MASTERING DIABETES

YOUR COMPLETE GUIDE TO LIVING WELL

TABLE OF CONTENTS

INTRODUCTION

- **Why This Book?**
    - Explain the purpose of the book, the need for comprehensive information on diabetes, and how it can help people manage their condition effectively.
- **Understanding Diabetes**
    - Overview of diabetes, including types (Type 1, Type 2, Gestational, and Prediabetes).
    - Importance of managing blood sugar levels and the impact on overall health.
    - Introduction to the key components of diabetes management: diet, exercise, medication, and lifestyle changes.

SECTION ONE: UNDERSTANDING DIABETES

Chapter 1: The Science Behind Diabetes

- **What is Diabetes?**
    - The role of insulin and glucose in the body.

- o Differences between Type 1, Type 2, Gestational Diabetes, and Prediabetes.
- **The Body's Response to Glucose**
  - o How glucose is processed in a healthy body vs. a diabetic body.
- **The Impact of Diabetes on the Body**
  - o How uncontrolled diabetes can affect organs and systems (heart, kidneys, nerves, eyes).

Chapter 2: Diagnosing Diabetes

- **Symptoms of Diabetes**
  - o Early signs to watch for and when to seek medical advice.
- **Diagnostic Tests**
  - o Fasting blood sugar, A1C, Oral Glucose Tolerance Test (OGTT), and others.
- **Understanding Your Diagnosis**
  - o Interpreting test results and what they mean for your health.

Chapter 3: Risk Factors and Prevention

- **Risk Factors for Type 1 and Type 2 Diabetes**
  - o Genetic, lifestyle, and environmental factors.
- **Prevention Strategies for Prediabetes**
  - o How to reduce the risk of developing Type 2 diabetes.

Chapter 4: Building Your Healthcare Team

- **The Role of Healthcare Providers**
  - Endocrinologists, dietitians, diabetes educators, and primary care physicians.
- **Collaborative Care**
  - How to work with your healthcare team to create a personalized management plan.

Chapter 5: Nutrition and Meal Planning

- **The Importance of Diet in Diabetes Management**
  - How food affects blood sugar levels.
- **Understanding Carbohydrates**
  - Simple vs. complex carbs, glycemic index, and portion control.
- **Meal Planning for Diabetics**
  - Creating balanced meals with the right mix of carbs, proteins, and fats.
- **Special Diets and Considerations**
  - Vegetarian, vegan, low-carb, and other dietary approaches.
- **Healthy Recipes and Cooking Tips**
  - Simple, diabetes-friendly recipes and cooking methods.

Chapter 8: Monitoring Blood Sugar Levels

- **Why Monitoring is Important**
  - Understanding the patterns in your blood sugar levels.
- **How to Monitor Blood Sugar**
  - Using glucose meters, continuous glucose monitors (CGMs), and keeping a log.
- **Interpreting Your Results**
  - What your readings mean and when to take action.
- **Advanced Monitoring Techniques**
  - Ketone testing, A1C monitoring, and other advanced tools.

SECTION THREE: LIVING WELL WITH DIABETES

Chapter 9: Managing Stress and Emotional Well-being

- **The Connection Between Stress and Blood Sugar**
  - How stress affects diabetes and blood sugar levels.
- **Stress Management Techniques**
  - Meditation, deep breathing, yoga, and other relaxation methods.
- **Coping with Diabetes-Related Stress**
  - Dealing with the emotional impact of diabetes and seeking support.

- **Building a Support System**

  - The importance of family, friends, and support groups.

- **Foot Care**

    - o Preventing foot complications and proper foot care routines.

- **Oral Health**

    - o The link between diabetes and gum disease and maintaining oral health.

Chapter 14: Innovations in Diabetes Care

- **Emerging Technologies**

    - o The latest in glucose monitoring, insulin delivery, and diabetes management apps.

- **The Future of Diabetes Treatment**

    - o Advances in research, potential cures, and new treatment options.

Chapter 15: Long-Term Health and Wellness

- **Healthy Aging with Diabetes**

    - o Strategies for maintaining health as you age.

- **Adapting Your Management Plan Over Time**

    - o Adjusting your plan as your needs change.

- **Staying Informed**

    - o Keeping up with the latest research, guidelines, and recommendations.

Final Thoughts

- **Empowerment Through Knowledge**
    - Encouragement to take control of your health and live well with diabetes.
- **The Importance of Ongoing Management**
    - Reinforcement of the need for continuous monitoring, adjustments, and self-care.

Appendices

- **Glossary of Terms**
- **Resources for Diabetics**
    - Websites, books, support groups, and organizations.
- **Diabetes Management Checklist**
    - Daily, weekly, and monthly tasks for managing diabetes.
- **30 Days Meal Plan**
    - A variety of meal plans tailored to different dietary needs and preferences.
- **Exercise Log Template**

o   A template to track physical activity and its impact on blood sugar levels.

References

- **Citations of Studies and Sources**
    - o   All research, studies, and expert opinions referenced throughout the book.

About the Author

- **Author Bio**
    - o   Information about the author's background, expertise, and motivation for writing the book.

INTRODUCTION

WHY THIS BOOK?

Welcome to *Mastering Diabetes: A Comprehensive Guide to Managing Blood Sugar and Living Well*. If you or someone you love has been diagnosed with diabetes, you might be feeling overwhelmed or unsure of where to begin in managing this condition. Diabetes is a serious, chronic illness that affects millions of people worldwide, but with the right knowledge and tools, you can live a fulfilling and healthy life despite the challenges it presents.

The purpose of this book is to provide a clear, in-depth guide that empowers you to take control of your diabetes management. Whether you are newly diagnosed, living with Type 1 or Type 2 diabetes, or even managing gestational diabetes or prediabetes, this book will equip you with the information and strategies needed to manage your blood sugar levels, prevent complications, and enhance your quality of life.

Diabetes is not just about managing blood sugar—it's about making informed choices about your health, your lifestyle, and your well-being. This book addresses every facet of living with diabetes, from understanding the disease and its symptoms to practical advice on diet, exercise, medication, and emotional well-being. With a focus on simple, actionable steps, this guide is here to offer support, build confidence, and help you navigate the complexities of diabetes management with clarity and success.

Diabetes is a chronic condition that affects how your body processes blood sugar (glucose). Glucose is an essential source of energy for your cells, and the hormone insulin is responsible for helping glucose enter the cells from the bloodstream. In diabetes, your body either doesn't produce enough insulin or can't effectively use the insulin it does produce. This leads to high blood sugar levels, which over time can cause serious health complications if not managed properly.

There are several types of diabetes, each with its own unique characteristics and causes:

- **Type 1 Diabetes**:

  Type 1 diabetes is an autoimmune condition where the body's immune system mistakenly attacks and destroys the insulin-producing cells in the pancreas. This results in little to no insulin production. People with Type 1 diabetes must rely on insulin injections or an insulin pump to manage their blood sugar levels. It is typically diagnosed in childhood or adolescence but can develop in adults as well.

- **Type 2 Diabetes**:

  Type 2 diabetes is the most common form and occurs when the body becomes resistant to insulin or the pancreas can't produce enough insulin to maintain normal blood sugar levels. This type of diabetes is strongly linked to lifestyle factors such as diet, physical inactivity, and being overweight. It is most commonly diagnosed in adults, though it is increasingly being seen in children and adolescents.

- **Gestational Diabetes**:

  Gestational diabetes occurs during pregnancy when a woman's body cannot produce enough insulin to meet the increased demands. Although it typically goes away after childbirth, women who experience gestational diabetes are at a higher risk of developing Type 2 diabetes later in life.

- **Prediabetes**:

  Prediabetes is a condition where blood sugar levels are higher than normal, but not high enough to be classified as Type 2 diabetes. It's a warning sign that diabetes could develop in the future. However, with lifestyle changes, prediabetes can often be reversed, preventing the onset of Type 2 diabetes.

THE IMPORTANCE OF MANAGING BLOOD SUGAR LEVELS

Managing your blood sugar levels is the key to preventing or delaying complications associated with diabetes. When blood sugar levels remain consistently high, it can damage blood vessels, nerves, and organs, leading to complications such as:

- **Heart Disease:**

  Diabetes increases the risk of heart disease and stroke. High blood sugar can lead to increased plaque build-up in the arteries, contributing to cardiovascular problems.

- **Kidney Damage (Diabetic Nephropathy):**

  Over time, high blood sugar can damage the kidneys' filtering system, leading to kidney disease or even kidney failure.

- **Nerve Damage (Neuropathy):**

  High blood sugar can damage nerves, especially in the extremities, leading to numbness, tingling, and pain. It can also affect digestive systems and sexual function.

- **Eye Damage (Diabetic Retinopathy):**

  Uncontrolled blood sugar levels can damage the blood vessels in the retina, leading to vision problems or even blindness.

- **Increased Risk of Infections:**

  High blood sugar can weaken the immune system, making the body more susceptible to infections.

By maintaining healthy blood sugar levels, you reduce your risk of these complications, and you also enhance your energy levels, mental clarity, and overall well-being.

KEY COMPONENTS OF DIABETES MANAGEMENT

Diabetes management is not just about monitoring your blood sugar levels, it also involves a combination of healthy lifestyle choices and medical care. The key components of managing diabetes effectively include:

- **Diet**:

  What you eat plays a central role in controlling blood sugar. A balanced, nutritious diet can help stabilize your blood sugar levels and prevent spikes and crashes. It's important to understand how different foods affect your blood sugar and how to make healthier food choices.

- **Exercise**:

  Regular physical activity is a powerful tool in managing diabetes. Exercise helps your body use insulin more efficiently, which in turn helps lower blood sugar levels. A combination of aerobic exercise (such as walking or swimming) and strength training can greatly improve insulin sensitivity.

- **Medication**:

  Depending on the type and severity of your diabetes, you may need medication to help control your blood sugar levels. This could include oral medications, insulin injections, or other types of treatments. Your doctor will work with you to determine the right medication plan for your needs.

- **Lifestyle Changes**:

  In addition to diet and exercise, managing diabetes involves making adjustments to your daily routine. This includes stress management, getting enough sleep, staying hydrated, and monitoring your blood sugar regularly. Lifestyle changes can significantly improve your quality of life and help you live a long, healthy life with diabetes.

Throughout this book, you will find practical advice, tips, and resources to help you understand and implement these components into your everyday life. Whether you are newly diagnosed or have been living with diabetes for years, this guide will provide you with the knowledge and confidence you need to effectively manage your condition.

Let's take the first step together in mastering diabetes and living your best life!

Section 1:

Understanding Diabetes

Chapter 1: The Science Behind Diabetes

What is Diabetes?

Diabetes is a chronic condition that affects how the body regulates blood sugar (glucose), which is a vital source of energy for the body's cells. When we eat, our bodies break down the carbohydrates in food into glucose, which then enters the bloodstream. Insulin, a hormone produced by the pancreas, helps move glucose from the bloodstream into the cells where it is used for energy.

In diabetes, there is a problem with insulin production or insulin action, resulting in elevated blood sugar levels, known as hyperglycemia. If left uncontrolled, high blood sugar can cause serious complications over time, affecting organs and systems in the body.

There are several types of diabetes, each with unique causes and mechanisms. Let's explore each one:

Types of Diabetes

- **Type 1 Diabetes:** Type 1 diabetes is an autoimmune condition where the body's immune system attacks and destroys the insulin-producing beta cells in the pancreas. As a result, people with Type 1 diabetes produce little to no insulin. Without insulin, glucose cannot enter cells, leading to high blood sugar levels. Type 1 diabetes is typically diagnosed in childhood or adolescence, although it can develop at any age. Individuals with Type 1 diabetes require insulin therapy for life to manage their blood sugar levels.

- **Type 2 Diabetes**: Type 2 diabetes occurs when the body becomes resistant to the effects of insulin or when the pancreas is unable to produce enough insulin to maintain normal blood sugar levels. Unlike Type 1 diabetes, where the body produces no insulin, people with Type 2 diabetes still produce insulin, but their cells do not respond to it as effectively. Type 2 diabetes is often linked to lifestyle factors such as poor diet, physical inactivity, and obesity. It is most commonly diagnosed in adults but is increasingly being seen in children, adolescents, and young adults. Type 2 diabetes can sometimes be managed with lifestyle changes and medication, though insulin therapy may be required in advanced stages.

- **Gestational Diabetes**: Gestational diabetes occurs during pregnancy and affects how the body processes glucose. During pregnancy, the placenta produces hormones that can make cells less sensitive to insulin, leading to higher blood sugar levels. In gestational diabetes, the pancreas cannot produce enough insulin to overcome this resistance, resulting in elevated blood sugar. While gestational diabetes typically resolves after childbirth, women who experience it are at a higher risk of developing Type 2 diabetes later in life.

- **Prediabetes**: Prediabetes is a condition where blood sugar levels are higher than normal, but not yet high enough to be diagnosed as Type 2 diabetes. People with prediabetes often experience insulin resistance, and if left unchecked, prediabetes can develop into full-blown Type 2 diabetes. However, with lifestyle changes such as a healthy diet, regular exercise, and weight loss, prediabetes can often be reversed.

THE ROLE OF INSULIN AND GLUCOSE IN THE BODY

In a healthy individual, insulin plays a critical role in maintaining normal blood sugar levels. Here's how the process works:

1. **Digestion**: After you eat, your digestive system breaks down carbohydrates into glucose, which enters the bloodstream.
2. **Insulin Release**: In response to the rising blood sugar levels, the pancreas releases insulin into the bloodstream.
3. **Glucose Transport**: Insulin acts as a "key" that unlocks the doors of cells, allowing glucose to enter and be used as energy.
4. **Storage of Excess Glucose**: Any excess glucose that is not immediately needed for energy is stored in the liver and muscles for later use.
5. **Regulation of Blood Sugar**: As cells absorb glucose, blood sugar levels begin to decrease. The pancreas detects this and reduces insulin production, maintaining balance.

In diabetes, however, there is a disruption in this process:

- **Type 1 Diabetes**: The body produces little or no insulin due to the destruction of pancreatic cells.
- **Type 2 Diabetes**: The body either does not produce enough insulin or the cells become resistant to insulin, making it difficult for glucose to enter the cells.
- **Gestational Diabetes**: Hormonal changes during pregnancy make it harder for the body to use insulin effectively, resulting in high blood sugar levels.

THE BODY'S RESPONSE TO GLUCOSE

Understanding how glucose is processed in a healthy body versus a diabetic body is essential in managing diabetes.

- **In a Healthy Body**:
  When you consume food, particularly carbohydrates, the glucose from digestion enters the bloodstream. The pancreas releases insulin in response to the elevated blood sugar levels, ensuring that glucose is taken up by cells for energy. This process keeps blood sugar levels within a narrow, healthy range (typically between 70-99 mg/dL when fasting).

- **In a Diabetic Body**:

  In individuals with diabetes, there is a breakdown in the regulation of blood sugar:

  - **Type 1 Diabetes**: The lack of insulin means glucose cannot enter the cells and accumulates in the bloodstream, leading to high blood sugar.
  - **Type 2 Diabetes**: The insulin resistance means cells don't respond to insulin properly, so glucose is not efficiently absorbed, and the pancreas must produce more insulin to compensate. Over time, the pancreas may not be able to keep up, leading to high blood sugar.
  - **Gestational Diabetes**: The body's increased insulin resistance during pregnancy leads to elevated blood sugar, but insulin production is often not sufficient to compensate.

In all forms of diabetes, the lack of proper glucose regulation can cause both short-term and long-term complications, which is why managing blood sugar levels is so critical.

THE IMPACT OF DIABETES ON THE BODY

Uncontrolled diabetes can affect various organs and systems in the body. Prolonged high blood sugar can lead to damage and dysfunction in the following areas:

- **Heart:**

  High blood sugar can increase the risk of cardiovascular diseases, including heart disease, stroke, and high blood pressure. Diabetes accelerates the buildup of plaque in the arteries (atherosclerosis), leading to reduced blood flow and increased strain on the heart.

- **Kidneys (Diabetic Nephropathy):**

  Over time, high blood sugar can damage the small blood vessels in the kidneys, impairing their ability to filter waste products and excess fluids. This condition, known as diabetic nephropathy, can eventually lead to kidney failure if not managed effectively.

- **Nerves (Neuropathy):**

  Chronic high blood sugar can damage the nerves, leading to diabetic neuropathy. This condition can cause numbness, tingling, pain, or weakness, especially in the extremities like the hands and feet. In severe cases, it can affect the digestive system, sexual function, and even lead to amputations due to poor circulation.

- **Eyes (Diabetic Retinopathy):**

  High blood sugar can damage the blood vessels in the retina, the light-sensitive layer at the back of the eye. Diabetic retinopathy can cause vision problems and, if left untreated, lead to blindness. Regular eye check-ups are essential for detecting and managing this complication.

By understanding the science behind diabetes and the impact it has on the body, you are better equipped to manage the condition and prevent complications. In the next chapters, we will delve into practical strategies for managing blood sugar, including diet, exercise, medication, and lifestyle changes.

CHAPTER 2: DIAGNOSING DIABETES

Symptoms of Diabetes

Early detection of diabetes is essential for effective management and to prevent complications. The symptoms of diabetes can develop gradually and may vary depending on the type of diabetes. Some individuals may not experience noticeable symptoms, especially in the early stages. However, here are common signs to watch for:

- **Increased Thirst (Polydipsia):** Excess sugar in the blood causes the kidneys to work harder to filter and absorb the excess glucose. This leads to dehydration, making you feel excessively thirsty.
- **Frequent Urination (Polyuria):** High blood sugar levels can lead to the kidneys filtering more urine, which results in frequent urination, especially during the night.
- **Fatigue:** When cells do not receive the glucose they need for energy due to insulin resistance or lack of insulin, it can cause feelings of extreme tiredness or fatigue.
- **Blurred Vision:** High blood sugar can lead to fluid being pulled from the lenses of the eyes, affecting your ability to focus and causing blurred vision.

- **Slow-Healing Sores and Frequent Infections**: Elevated blood sugar levels impair the immune system, making it harder for the body to fight infections and heal wounds.

- **Unexplained Weight Loss**: In Type 1 diabetes, the body cannot use glucose for energy due to lack of insulin, leading to muscle and fat breakdown for energy. This can result in significant weight loss despite normal or increased food intake.

- **Increased Hunger (Polyphagia)**: Without enough insulin, the body's cells cannot absorb glucose properly, which can lead to an increase in hunger as the body seeks more energy sources.

- **Tingling or Numbness in Hands or Feet**: High blood sugar levels can damage the nerves, leading to neuropathy, which may cause a tingling, numbness, or burning sensation, particularly in the hands and feet.

If you experience any of these symptoms, it is important to consult a healthcare provider for further evaluation. Early diagnosis and management are critical to controlling blood sugar and reducing the risk of complications.

Diagnostic Tests

There are several tests used to diagnose diabetes and prediabetes. These tests measure the amount of glucose in the blood and provide valuable information for diagnosis and management. Below are the most common diagnostic tests:

- **Fasting Blood Sugar (FBS)**:

  This test measures blood glucose levels after an overnight fast (usually 8-12 hours without food or drink). The results are categorized as follows:

  - Normal: Below 100 mg/dL
  - Prediabetes: 100-125 mg/dL
  - Diabetes: 126 mg/dL or higher (on two separate tests)

- **Hemoglobin A1C (HbA1C)**:

  The A1C test measures the average blood glucose levels over the past 2-3 months by assessing the percentage of hemoglobin in the blood that has glucose attached to it. It provides a long-term view of blood sugar control. The results are interpreted as:

  - Normal: Below 5.7%
  - Prediabetes: 5.7% - 6.4%
  - Diabetes: 6.5% or higher

  This test does not require fasting and is often used to monitor ongoing blood sugar control in diagnosed individuals.

- **Oral Glucose Tolerance Test (OGTT)**:

  This test involves fasting overnight and then drinking a sugary solution. Blood glucose levels are measured two hours later to see how the body processes glucose. This test is often used to diagnose gestational diabetes or confirm Type 2 diabetes:

- Normal: Less than 140 mg/dL

  - Prediabetes: 140-199 mg/dL

  - Diabetes: 200 mg/dL or higher

- **Random Blood Sugar Test:**

  A blood sample is taken at any time of the day, regardless of when you last ate. If the blood sugar level is 200 mg/dL or higher, diabetes may be diagnosed, especially if accompanied by symptoms like frequent urination and excessive thirst.

- **C-Peptide Test:**

  This test measures the level of C-peptide, which is a byproduct of insulin production. It can help distinguish between Type 1 and Type 2 diabetes. In Type 1 diabetes, C-peptide levels are usually low, while in Type 2 diabetes, they may be normal or high due to insulin resistance.

UNDERSTANDING YOUR DIAGNOSIS

Once diagnosed, it's important to interpret your test results and understand what they mean for your health. Here's a breakdown of what different results may indicate:

- **Normal Blood Sugar Levels:**

  - A normal blood sugar range (fasting below 100 mg/dL and A1C below 5.7%) indicates healthy blood sugar regulation.

Maintaining these levels through a balanced diet, exercise, and regular health check-ups can help prevent the onset of diabetes.

- **Prediabetes**:
    - Prediabetes is a condition where blood sugar levels are higher than normal but not yet high enough to be classified as diabetes. It is a warning sign and an opportunity to reverse the condition through lifestyle changes. The goal is to bring blood sugar levels back to normal through a healthy diet, increased physical activity, and weight management.

- **Diabetes**:
    - A diagnosis of diabetes means that your blood sugar levels are consistently elevated, and your body is not managing glucose effectively. In Type 1 diabetes, your pancreas is not producing insulin, while in Type 2 diabetes, your cells are not responding properly to insulin. Gestational diabetes typically resolves after pregnancy, but it requires careful management during and after pregnancy to prevent complications. People with diabetes must work with their healthcare provider to create a comprehensive management plan involving diet, exercise, and medication.

The A1C test is also an important tool for understanding long-term blood sugar control. Higher A1C levels indicate a higher risk of complications such as heart disease, kidney problems, neuropathy, and eye issues. Regular monitoring and adjustments to your treatment plan are essential to maintain optimal blood sugar control.

If you experience symptoms of diabetes or have risk factors such as a family history, obesity, or an inactive lifestyle, seek medical advice promptly. Early intervention can help prevent or delay the onset of Type 2 diabetes and improve management of Type 1 diabetes.

Additionally, if you are already diagnosed with diabetes, regular check-ups are crucial to monitor blood sugar levels, manage complications, and adjust treatment plans as needed. Working closely with your healthcare team, including a diabetes educator, dietitian, and endocrinologist, can help you achieve the best possible outcomes for your health.

Understanding your diagnosis is a key step toward effectively managing diabetes. In the next chapter, we will explore the fundamentals of managing blood sugar through diet, exercise, and medication.

CHAPTER 3: RISK FACTORS AND PREVENTION

Risk Factors for Type 1 and Type 2 Diabetes

Diabetes is a complex condition influenced by a combination of genetic, lifestyle, and environmental factors. While Type 1 and Type 2 diabetes have distinct causes, several overlapping risk factors exist. Understanding these risk factors can help in early identification and prevention.

Risk Factors for Type 1 Diabetes

Type 1 diabetes (T1D) is an autoimmune condition where the body's immune system mistakenly attacks the insulin-producing beta cells in the pancreas. The exact cause is not entirely understood, but several factors may increase the risk:

- **Genetic Factors**:
  Having a family history of Type 1 diabetes increases the risk. Certain genetic markers, such as those found on the HLA (human leukocyte antigen) gene, are linked to an increased risk of developing the condition. However, not everyone with these markers will develop Type 1 diabetes, indicating other environmental factors are involved.

- **Autoimmune Response:**

  Type 1 diabetes is often triggered by an autoimmune response, where the immune system attacks the beta cells in the pancreas. This can occur following viral infections, though the exact viruses that may trigger this immune response are still being studied.

- **Age:**

  Type 1 diabetes is most commonly diagnosed in children, adolescents, and young adults, but it can develop at any age.

- **Geography and Ethnicity:**

  Type 1 diabetes is more common in countries with colder climates, and it has a higher prevalence in people of European descent compared to other ethnic groups.

- **Environmental Factors:**

  Exposure to certain viruses or toxins might trigger an autoimmune response in individuals genetically predisposed to Type 1 diabetes, although the specific triggers remain uncertain.

RISK FACTORS FOR TYPE 2 DIABETES

Type 2 diabetes (T2D) is primarily a condition of insulin resistance, where the body's cells do not respond properly to insulin, leading to high blood sugar levels. It is a multifactorial condition, and several risk factors are associated with its development:

- **Age**:

  The risk of developing Type 2 diabetes increases with age, especially after age 45. This is partly due to natural changes in metabolism and insulin sensitivity as people age.

- **Family History and Genetics**:

  A family history of Type 2 diabetes significantly increases the risk of developing the condition. If your parents or siblings have Type 2 diabetes, your risk is higher. Certain genetic variations also predispose individuals to Type 2 diabetes.

- **Obesity and Overweight**:

  Excess body fat, especially abdominal fat, is a major risk factor for insulin resistance. The more overweight you are, the more likely your body is to develop insulin resistance, which can lead to Type 2 diabetes.

- **Physical Inactivity**:

  A sedentary lifestyle is a major contributing factor to the development of Type 2 diabetes. Regular physical activity helps the body use insulin more effectively and reduces blood sugar levels.

- **Unhealthy Diet**:

  Diets high in refined carbohydrates, sugary foods, and unhealthy fats can contribute to the development of Type 2 diabetes. A lack of fiber and nutrients in the diet can also affect insulin sensitivity and blood sugar control.

- **High Blood Pressure and Cholesterol**:

High blood pressure and abnormal cholesterol levels are common in people with Type 2 diabetes and can contribute to complications. Insulin resistance is often linked to these conditions.

- **Gestational Diabetes**:

Women who have had gestational diabetes during pregnancy are at higher risk of developing Type 2 diabetes later in life. The condition also increases the risk of the baby developing Type 2 diabetes in the future.

- **Ethnicity**:

Type 2 diabetes is more common in certain ethnic groups, including African Americans, Hispanic Americans, Native Americans, and Asian Americans. Genetic factors and lifestyle choices are believed to contribute to this increased risk.

- **Polycystic Ovary Syndrome (PCOS)**:

Women with PCOS are at higher risk of developing insulin resistance, which can lead to Type 2 diabetes. PCOS is often associated with obesity and hormonal imbalances that contribute to insulin resistance.

Prediabetes is a condition where blood sugar levels are higher than normal but not yet high enough to be classified as diabetes. It is an important warning sign that should not be ignored, as it can progress to Type 2 diabetes if not addressed. Fortunately, lifestyle changes can help reverse prediabetes and prevent the onset of Type 2 diabetes. Here are key prevention strategies:

---

1. HEALTHY DIET

Adopting a balanced diet is one of the most effective ways to prevent the progression of prediabetes. Focus on:

- **Whole Grains**: Opt for whole grains instead of refined carbs (such as white bread and pasta). Whole grains help improve insulin sensitivity and are rich in fiber, which helps stabilize blood sugar levels.
- **Fiber-Rich Foods**: Incorporate plenty of vegetables, fruits, and legumes, as fiber slows the absorption of glucose and helps maintain healthy blood sugar levels.
- **Healthy Fats**: Include unsaturated fats like those from avocados, olive oil, nuts, and seeds, which can help improve insulin sensitivity.

- **Protein**: Choose lean protein sources such as poultry, fish, and plant-based proteins (tofu, legumes, etc.), which help regulate blood sugar without causing spikes.

- **Portion Control**: Managing portion sizes helps prevent overeating and keeps blood sugar levels stable.

- **Limit Sugar and Processed Foods**: Avoid sugary drinks, snacks, and processed foods, as they can cause rapid spikes in blood sugar levels and contribute to insulin resistance.

---

2. REGULAR PHYSICAL ACTIVITY

Exercise is essential for preventing and managing prediabetes. It helps lower blood sugar levels, increases insulin sensitivity, and supports weight management. Aim for:

- **Aerobic Exercise**: Activities like walking, jogging, swimming, or cycling can help improve cardiovascular health and insulin sensitivity.

- **Strength Training**: Incorporating resistance exercises such as weightlifting or bodyweight exercises helps build muscle, which in turn improves glucose metabolism.

- **Consistency**: Aim for at least 150 minutes of moderate-intensity aerobic activity per week (such as brisk walking) and strength training exercises twice a week.

3. Weight Loss

If you're overweight or obese, even a modest weight loss of 5-10% of your body weight can significantly reduce your risk of developing Type 2 diabetes. Focus on:

- **Gradual Weight Loss**: Rapid weight loss can be unsustainable and unhealthy. Aim for gradual weight loss through a combination of diet and exercise.
- **Healthy Habits**: Focus on long-term lifestyle changes such as adopting healthy eating patterns and increasing physical activity rather than quick-fix diets.

4. Monitor Blood Sugar Levels

If you have prediabetes, it's important to monitor your blood sugar levels regularly. This helps you track changes and see if your lifestyle changes are effectively managing your glucose levels.

5. Get Regular Check-ups

Regular visits to your healthcare provider allow for early detection of any changes in your blood sugar levels and provide an opportunity to make adjustments to your management plan. Your provider can also guide you on how to manage any other health conditions that may increase your risk of diabetes.

---

6. REDUCE STRESS

Chronic stress can increase blood sugar levels and contribute to insulin resistance. Stress-reducing activities such as mindfulness, yoga, and meditation can help lower stress and improve overall health.

---

7. GET ENOUGH SLEEP

Poor sleep quality and insufficient sleep have been linked to insulin resistance and an increased risk of developing Type 2 diabetes. Aim for 7-9 hours of quality sleep each night to help regulate your blood sugar levels and support overall well-being.

CONCLUSION

While the risk factors for diabetes vary between Type 1 and Type 2 diabetes, there are clear steps you can take to reduce the risk of developing Type 2 diabetes and manage prediabetes. Adopting a healthy diet, engaging in regular physical activity, maintaining a healthy weight, and reducing stress are crucial steps in preventing the progression of prediabetes to Type 2 diabetes. With proper lifestyle changes and regular check-ups, you can take control of your health and prevent diabetes-related complications.

In the next chapter, we will dive deeper into the specific dietary and lifestyle strategies that can help you manage diabetes effectively.

SECTION 2:

DEVELOPING A DIABETES MANAGEMENT PLAN

Chapter 4: Building Your Healthcare Team

Managing diabetes requires a comprehensive approach, and having the right healthcare team can make a significant difference in how effectively you manage the condition. Diabetes care is multifaceted, involving medication, lifestyle changes, and monitoring of blood sugar levels. The collaboration of various healthcare professionals ensures that all aspects of diabetes management are covered. In this chapter, we will discuss the roles of key healthcare providers and how to collaborate with them to build a personalized diabetes management plan.

The Role of Healthcare Providers

When it comes to managing diabetes, you'll likely work with a variety of healthcare professionals. Each has a unique role in your care, and working closely with them can help ensure the best outcomes for your health.

Endocrinologists

An **endocrinologist** is a medical doctor who specializes in hormone-related conditions, including diabetes. They are experts in managing both Type 1 and Type 2 diabetes, and their role is particularly important for individuals with more complex or advanced cases of diabetes. They will:

- **Diagnose and treat diabetes**: They can determine the type of diabetes and help manage more complicated cases that may involve hormonal imbalances or other endocrine-related conditions.
- **Provide insulin and medication management**: Endocrinologists have extensive knowledge of the various diabetes medications available, including insulin therapy, oral medications, and newer treatments. They will help you understand your medications and how to use them effectively.
- **Monitor long-term complications**: Since diabetes can lead to complications affecting the heart, kidneys, eyes, and nerves, endocrinologists will monitor these areas and provide advice on how to manage or prevent them.

PRIMARY CARE PHYSICIANS (PCPS)

Your **primary care physician** is the first point of contact for general health concerns. They will help with initial diagnosis, basic diabetes management, and referrals to specialists when needed. The PCP's role includes:

- **Routine check-ups and monitoring**: They will regularly check your blood pressure, cholesterol levels, and kidney function to ensure that your diabetes is being well-managed.
- **Medication management**: For people with Type 2 diabetes, a PCP may prescribe oral medications and offer lifestyle advice.

- **General health maintenance**: Your PCP will coordinate with other specialists and help manage other health conditions, such as high blood pressure or high cholesterol, that may complicate diabetes.

DIETITIANS

A **dietitian** (often a registered dietitian nutritionist, or RDN) is an expert in nutrition and helps design a personalized meal plan that suits your needs. Since diet plays a critical role in diabetes management, a dietitian will:

- **Help design a balanced meal plan**: They will work with you to develop a meal plan that controls blood sugar levels, promotes healthy weight management, and meets your dietary preferences.
- **Teach about carbohydrate counting**: Understanding how to manage carbohydrate intake is essential for blood sugar control. A dietitian will guide you on how to count carbs, balance meals, and understand how different foods impact your blood sugar.
- **Monitor nutritional needs**: People with diabetes may have specific nutritional needs that need to be addressed, such as ensuring proper intake of fiber, vitamins, and minerals, as well as monitoring kidney function and reducing salt intake.

Diabetes educators are healthcare professionals who specialize in teaching people with diabetes about the condition and how to manage it. Their role is to empower you with knowledge and practical skills, including:

- **Blood sugar monitoring**: Diabetes educators will teach you how to measure your blood sugar levels, interpret the results, and make adjustments to your diet, exercise, or medication accordingly.
- **Insulin administration**: If you're on insulin therapy, they will provide hands-on training on how to inject insulin properly, including understanding dosages and timing.
- **Behavioral change**: They can guide you in making healthy lifestyle changes, such as adopting a balanced diet, incorporating exercise, and coping with the emotional aspects of living with diabetes.

OTHER SPECIALISTS

Depending on your specific health needs, other specialists might become involved in your diabetes care:

- **Cardiologists**: If you have diabetes-related heart issues or other cardiovascular conditions, a cardiologist will monitor and manage those aspects.

- **Ophthalmologists**: Regular eye exams are crucial for people with diabetes, as high blood sugar can cause eye problems, including diabetic retinopathy.
- **Podiatrists**: Diabetes can affect foot health, so seeing a podiatrist regularly can help prevent complications such as infections or ulcers.
- **Nephrologists**: If diabetes affects your kidneys, a nephrologist will help manage kidney health and any early signs of diabetic nephropathy.

COLLABORATIVE CARE: BUILDING A PERSONALIZED MANAGEMENT PLAN

Having a team of healthcare providers can seem overwhelming, but with the right approach, it can be an incredibly powerful tool in managing your diabetes. Collaborative care is about working together with your team to create a comprehensive, individualized management plan that addresses your specific health needs and goals.

1. OPEN COMMUNICATION

The foundation of successful diabetes management is open, honest communication. Be sure to share all relevant information with your healthcare providers, including:

- **Symptoms**: Report any changes in your health, even if they seem minor. New symptoms might indicate a need for adjustments in your management plan.
- **Medications**: Inform your healthcare providers of all the medications you are taking, including over-the-counter drugs, supplements, and herbal remedies, as they can interact with diabetes medications.
- **Lifestyle**: Share your daily routines, including diet, exercise, work, and sleep habits, so your team can help tailor a plan that fits your lifestyle.
- **Goals and Preferences**: Your healthcare team should understand your personal goals for managing diabetes, whether it's weight loss, managing stress, or improving blood sugar levels.

2. REGULAR CHECK-INS

Managing diabetes is a long-term commitment. Regular visits with your healthcare team are crucial for adjusting treatment plans and tracking progress. These visits may include:

- **Regular blood tests**: Blood sugar levels, A1C, cholesterol, and kidney function should be tested regularly to monitor your condition and adjust treatment.
- **Progress evaluations**: Your healthcare providers will assess how well your diabetes management plan is working, including any changes in your lifestyle, diet, and medication.

3. Education and Self-Management

Diabetes is a condition that requires active participation from you, the patient. A large part of effective management is learning how to care for yourself, which involves:

- **Self-monitoring of blood glucose**: Learning how to monitor your blood sugar levels is essential. Your healthcare provider or diabetes educator will guide you on how to interpret your results and take action when needed.
- **Understanding your medications**: Learn about your diabetes medications, how they work, and how they affect your blood sugar. Your healthcare team can help you understand the importance of taking medications as prescribed and discuss potential side effects.
- **Behavioral changes**: Your healthcare team will assist you in developing long-term, sustainable changes to your diet, exercise, and stress management habits.

4. Tailored Support

Each person with diabetes has unique needs and challenges. Working with a collaborative team allows for a personalized approach to diabetes management. Whether you need extra support managing stress, dietary advice, or help with medication adherence, your team can provide customized solutions to meet your goals.

CONCLUSION

Building a strong healthcare team is essential in managing diabetes. With professionals like endocrinologists, dietitians, diabetes educators, and your primary care physician, you can create a comprehensive, personalized plan that addresses all aspects of your health. By communicating openly, staying engaged in your care, and collaborating with your healthcare providers, you can successfully manage your diabetes and reduce the risk of complications. In the next chapter, we will explore how to design a daily management routine that fits your lifestyle and helps maintain stable blood sugar levels.

Chapter 5: Nutrition and Meal Planning

One of the most important aspects of managing diabetes is maintaining a balanced and healthy diet. The food you eat directly impacts your blood sugar levels, which in turn affects your overall health. By understanding how different foods affect your body and learning how to plan your meals effectively, you can achieve better blood sugar control, prevent complications, and improve your quality of life. In this chapter, we will explore the importance of diet in diabetes management, break down carbohydrates and their impact on blood sugar, and provide practical meal planning tips and healthy recipes tailored for those living with diabetes.

The Importance of Diet in Diabetes Management

Diet plays a central role in managing diabetes. When you have diabetes, your body either does not produce enough insulin (in the case of Type 1 diabetes) or does not respond effectively to insulin (in the case of Type 2 diabetes). As a result, the food you consume—especially carbohydrates—has a significant impact on your blood sugar levels.

Why Food Matters:

- **Blood Sugar Control**: Carbohydrates are broken down into glucose (sugar) in the body, which raises blood sugar levels. The key to managing diabetes is controlling how much glucose enters the bloodstream, and diet is the primary way to achieve this.
- **Preventing Complications**: Proper nutrition can help prevent or delay complications related to diabetes, including heart disease, kidney failure, nerve damage, and vision loss.
- **Overall Health**: A well-balanced diet not only helps manage blood sugar but also supports your cardiovascular health, weight management, and general well-being.

By following a healthy eating plan, you can improve your insulin sensitivity, control your blood sugar, and reduce your risk of complications.

UNDERSTANDING CARBOHYDRATES

Carbohydrates are the main nutrient that affects blood sugar levels, so it is crucial to understand how they work. All carbohydrates eventually turn into glucose in the body, but not all carbs have the same effect on blood sugar.

SIMPLE VS. COMPLEX CARBOHYDRATES

- **Simple Carbohydrates**: These are quickly digested and cause a rapid spike in blood sugar. They are found in foods like candy, soda, baked goods, and other processed foods. Simple carbs are generally low in fiber and nutrients.

- o *Examples*: Table sugar, syrups, candy, sugary drinks, and refined grains (white bread, white rice, pasta).
- **Complex Carbohydrates**: These are digested more slowly and have a gentler effect on blood sugar. They are found in whole grains, vegetables, legumes, and fruits. Complex carbs are usually rich in fiber, which helps control blood sugar levels and supports digestive health.
  - o *Examples*: Whole grains (brown rice, quinoa, whole wheat), legumes (beans, lentils), vegetables (broccoli, spinach), and fruits (berries, apples).

FIBER AND CARBOHYDRATE CONTROL:

- Fiber, found in complex carbohydrates, helps slow down the digestion and absorption of sugar, which can prevent sharp blood sugar spikes. Focus on incorporating fiber-rich foods into your diet to improve blood sugar control.

GLYCEMIC INDEX (GI) AND GLYCEMIC LOAD (GL)

- **Glycemic Index (GI)** measures how quickly a carbohydrate-containing food raises blood sugar levels. Foods with a high GI (like white bread and sugary snacks) are quickly broken down into glucose, while foods with a low GI (like whole grains and legumes) are digested more slowly.

- **Glycemic Load (GL)** takes into account both the glycemic index of a food and the amount of carbohydrate in a typical serving. It is a better indicator of how a food will affect blood sugar levels.

GLYCEMIC INDEX CHART:

- Low GI foods: Whole grains, legumes, non-starchy vegetables, and most fruits (apples, berries, oranges).
- High GI foods: Refined grains (white bread, white rice), sugary cereals, and processed snacks.

Understanding the glycemic index and glycemic load can help you make smarter food choices and keep your blood sugar stable.

MEAL PLANNING FOR DIABETICS

Effective meal planning is essential for diabetes management. By creating balanced meals with the right mix of carbohydrates, proteins, and fats, you can maintain steady blood sugar levels throughout the day.

THE THREE MACRONUTRIENTS:

- **Carbohydrates**: Aim to get your carbs primarily from whole, fiber-rich foods such as vegetables, fruits, whole grains, and legumes. Limit your intake of processed and sugary foods.

- **Proteins**: Proteins help stabilize blood sugar levels and provide long-lasting energy. Include lean protein sources like poultry, fish, eggs, tofu, and legumes.

- **Fats**: Healthy fats, such as those found in avocados, nuts, seeds, and olive oil, promote satiety, stabilize blood sugar levels, and support overall health. Focus on unsaturated fats while minimizing trans fats and saturated fats.

BUILDING BALANCED MEALS:

A good rule of thumb for meal planning is the "plate method," which divides your plate into sections for each food group:

- **Half the plate**: Non-starchy vegetables (e.g., spinach, broccoli, cauliflower, bell peppers).

- **One-quarter of the plate**: Lean protein (e.g., chicken, fish, tofu, eggs).

- **One-quarter of the plate**: Carbohydrates (e.g., brown rice, quinoa, sweet potatoes, whole wheat pasta).

- **Include healthy fats**: Add a small amount of olive oil, avocado, or nuts to your meals.

- **Meal Timing**: Eating regular, balanced meals throughout the day helps keep blood sugar levels steady. Avoid skipping meals, as it can cause blood sugar fluctuations.
- **Portion Control**: Even healthy foods can contribute to high blood sugar if eaten in large quantities. Learn to control portion sizes, particularly with carbohydrate-rich foods.

SPECIAL DIETS AND CONSIDERATIONS

While there is no one-size-fits-all diet for diabetes, certain dietary approaches can be beneficial depending on your health goals, preferences, and lifestyle.

Vegetarian or Vegan Diet

A vegetarian or vegan diet can be a healthy option for people with diabetes, as long as it includes a variety of plant-based foods that are high in fiber and protein. Be mindful of:

- **Carbohydrate quality**: Focus on whole grains, legumes, and non-starchy vegetables.
- **Protein sources**: Include beans, lentils, tofu, tempeh, and seitan for adequate protein.

- **Iron and B12**: Vegetarians and vegans need to ensure adequate intake of iron and B12, which are found in animal products.

Low-Carb Diet

Some people with diabetes find that a low-carbohydrate diet helps with blood sugar control. This approach typically involves reducing intake of bread, pasta, rice, and sugary foods. However, it's important to focus on **healthy carbs** such as non-starchy vegetables, legumes, and whole grains to maintain fiber intake.

Mediterranean Diet

The Mediterranean diet emphasizes whole grains, lean proteins (such as fish), healthy fats (like olive oil), and plenty of fruits and vegetables. It has been shown to help manage blood sugar levels and reduce the risk of heart disease, which is important for people with diabetes.

Healthy Recipes and Cooking Tips

Creating diabetes-friendly meals doesn't have to be complicated or bland. Here are some simple recipes and cooking tips to get you started:

- **Ingredients**: 1/2 cup rolled oats, 1 cup unsweetened almond milk, 1/4 cup fresh berries (blueberries, strawberries), 1 tablespoon chopped almonds, cinnamon.
- **Directions**: Cook the oats with almond milk over medium heat until soft. Top with berries, almonds, and a sprinkle of cinnamon for flavor.
- **Why It's Healthy**: Oats are a whole grain and a great source of soluble fiber, which helps control blood sugar levels. Berries provide antioxidants and a touch of natural sweetness.

LUNCH: GRILLED CHICKEN SALAD WITH AVOCADO

- **Ingredients**: 4 oz grilled chicken breast, mixed greens (spinach, kale, arugula), 1/2 avocado, cherry tomatoes, cucumber, olive oil and balsamic vinegar dressing.
- **Directions**: Toss all ingredients in a large bowl and drizzle with olive oil and vinegar dressing.
- **Why It's Healthy**: This salad is rich in lean protein, healthy fats, and fiber, all of which help stabilize blood sugar.

DINNER: BAKED SALMON WITH QUINOA AND ROASTED VEGETABLES

- **Ingredients**: 4 oz salmon fillet, 1/2 cup cooked quinoa, 1 cup mixed vegetables (broccoli, carrots, zucchini), olive oil, garlic, lemon.

- **Directions**: Bake the salmon with a drizzle of olive oil, garlic, and lemon at 375°F for 15-20 minutes. Roast the vegetables in the oven at the same time. Serve with quinoa.
- **Why It's Healthy**: Salmon is a great source of omega-3 fatty acids, which are heart-healthy. Quinoa provides fiber and protein, and the vegetables add a variety of nutrients.

CONCLUSION

Nutrition is a cornerstone of diabetes management. By understanding how food affects your blood sugar and learning to plan balanced meals, you can take control of your health and improve your quality of life. Whether you choose a vegetarian, low-carb, or Mediterranean approach, the key is to focus on whole, nutrient-dense foods and portion control. With careful planning and the right support, managing your diabetes through diet can become a sustainable and empowering part of your daily routine. In the next chapter, we will explore how to incorporate exercise into your diabetes management plan.

Chapter 6: Exercise and Physical Activity

Exercise is one of the most effective ways to manage diabetes and improve overall health. Regular physical activity not only helps control blood sugar levels but also reduces the risk of complications such as heart disease, nerve damage, and high blood pressure. It can improve insulin sensitivity, help with weight management, and promote mental well-being. In this chapter, we will explore the role of exercise in diabetes management, the different types of exercise that benefit those with diabetes, how to create a personalized exercise routine, and how to stay motivated to stay active.

The Role of Exercise in Diabetes Management

Physical activity plays a crucial role in managing diabetes for several reasons:

1. **Improves Insulin Sensitivity**: Exercise helps your body use insulin more effectively, which can reduce the amount of insulin needed to control blood sugar levels.
2. **Regulates Blood Sugar**: Both aerobic and strength exercises can help lower blood glucose levels, especially after meals, by encouraging the muscles to take in glucose for energy.

3. **Weight Management**: Maintaining a healthy weight is vital for diabetes control. Regular exercise, combined with a balanced diet, can help you lose excess weight or maintain a healthy weight.

4. **Reduces Cardiovascular Risk**: People with diabetes are at an increased risk for heart disease. Exercise helps reduce this risk by improving cholesterol levels, lowering blood pressure, and improving circulation.

5. **Improves Mental Health**: Exercise can reduce stress, anxiety, and depression—common challenges for people living with diabetes. It can also improve sleep quality, which is crucial for overall health.

By incorporating exercise into your daily routine, you can take a proactive approach to managing your diabetes and enhance your quality of life.

TYPES OF EXERCISE

There are several types of exercise that can benefit people with diabetes. Each type offers unique benefits and can help you achieve different health goals. It's important to incorporate a variety of exercises to keep your routine balanced and engaging.

1. Aerobic Exercise

Aerobic exercise is any activity that raises your heart rate and helps improve cardiovascular health. It also helps the body use insulin more effectively, which can lower blood sugar levels.

- **Examples**: Walking, jogging, cycling, swimming, dancing, and using machines like a treadmill, elliptical, or stationary bike.
- **Benefits**: Improves heart health, helps with weight management, lowers blood sugar, boosts energy levels.
- **Recommendation**: Aim for at least 150 minutes of moderate-intensity aerobic exercise per week, or 75 minutes of vigorous activity spread throughout the week.

2. STRENGTH TRAINING

Strength training (also known as resistance or weight training) involves exercises that build muscle mass. It is especially important for people with Type 2 diabetes, as it helps improve insulin sensitivity and regulate blood sugar levels over time.

- **Examples**: Weightlifting, bodyweight exercises (squats, lunges, push-ups), resistance bands, or using gym equipment like machines.
- **Benefits**: Builds muscle mass, which increases the amount of glucose your muscles can absorb; improves blood sugar control; enhances metabolism and fat burning.

- **Recommendation**: Aim for two to three strength training sessions per week, focusing on all major muscle groups.

3. FLEXIBILITY EXERCISES

Flexibility exercises help improve the range of motion in your joints and muscles. While they may not directly affect blood sugar, they help prevent injuries and improve overall physical function.

- **Examples**: Yoga, Pilates, stretching routines, tai chi.
- **Benefits**: Enhances joint mobility, reduces muscle stiffness, improves balance and posture, promotes relaxation and stress reduction.
- **Recommendation**: Incorporate flexibility exercises into your routine 2-3 times per week.

4. BALANCE EXERCISES

Balance exercises are essential for preventing falls and improving stability, especially as we age. They are especially beneficial for people with diabetes who may experience nerve damage (neuropathy) that affects balance.

- **Examples**: Standing on one leg, heel-to-toe walking, balance board exercises, and certain yoga poses.
- **Benefits**: Improves coordination, strengthens muscles involved in balance, reduces fall risk, and enhances overall mobility.

- **Recommendation**: Perform balance exercises 2-3 times a week, focusing on improving stability and coordination.

CREATING AN EXERCISE ROUTINE

Creating a personalized exercise routine is key to ensuring that you stay active, avoid injury, and reap the full benefits of physical activity. Your exercise plan should be tailored to your fitness level, preferences, and goals.

1. START SLOWLY AND BUILD UP

If you're new to exercise, it's important to start slow and gradually increase the intensity and duration of your workouts. Begin with shorter sessions (15-20 minutes) of moderate-intensity aerobic exercise and work your way up to 30 minutes or more. As you gain strength and endurance, you can incorporate more intense workouts.

2. SET REALISTIC GOALS

Set achievable and measurable fitness goals, such as walking for 30 minutes every day, lifting weights twice a week, or completing a specific number of steps each day. This helps keep you motivated and gives you a sense of accomplishment.

3. COMBINE DIFFERENT TYPES OF EXERCISE

For maximum benefits, aim to include a mix of aerobic exercise, strength training, and flexibility/balance exercises into your routine. For example, you could walk briskly on Mondays, do strength training on Wednesdays, and practice yoga on Fridays.

4. LISTEN TO YOUR BODY

Pay attention to how your body responds to exercise. If you experience pain, dizziness, or shortness of breath, stop and consult your healthcare provider before continuing. It's important to exercise at a pace that feels comfortable but still challenges you.

5. MAKE EXERCISE A HABIT

Consistency is key. Try to schedule your workouts at the same time each day, making them a non-negotiable part of your daily routine. You can also exercise with a friend or family member to make it more enjoyable.

STAYING MOTIVATED

Maintaining an active lifestyle can be challenging, especially when you're juggling other responsibilities. However, staying motivated is crucial for long-term success in diabetes management. Here are some tips to help you stay on track:

1. FIND ACTIVITIES YOU ENJOY

Choose exercises that you like and look forward to. If you hate running, try cycling or dancing instead. Engaging in activities that bring you joy makes it easier to stay consistent.

2. TRACK YOUR PROGRESS

Keep a log of your physical activity to track your progress. Write down the duration, intensity, and how you felt after each workout. Over time, you'll see improvements in your endurance, strength, and blood sugar control, which will keep you motivated.

3. REWARD YOURSELF

Celebrate your successes, no matter how small. After reaching a fitness goal, reward yourself with something you enjoy, such as a relaxing activity, new workout gear, or a favorite healthy meal.

4. Exercise with Others

Social support can be a powerful motivator. Find an exercise buddy, join a fitness class, or participate in community events like charity walks or runs. Exercising with others adds a sense of accountability and fun.

5. Make It Part of Your Lifestyle

Think of exercise as an integral part of your daily routine, just like brushing your teeth. When exercise becomes a habit, you're more likely to stick with it over the long term.

Conclusion

Exercise is a vital part of diabetes management and can significantly improve your quality of life. By incorporating a mix of aerobic, strength, flexibility, and balance exercises into your routine, you can lower your blood sugar levels, reduce the risk of complications, and improve your physical and mental health. Remember to start slowly, set realistic goals, and choose activities that you enjoy. With consistency and dedication, you can maintain an active lifestyle that supports your diabetes management and overall well-being. In the next chapter, we will explore medication and insulin management for people with diabetes.

Chapter 7: Medication Management

Managing diabetes effectively often requires medication, especially when lifestyle changes alone are not enough to control blood sugar levels. Medications play a crucial role in managing both Type 1 and Type 2 diabetes. Whether you're prescribed oral medications, insulin, or other injectables, understanding how these medications work, their side effects, and how to manage them is vital for maintaining good blood sugar control and overall health. In this chapter, we will explore the types of diabetes medications, how they work, insulin therapy, and strategies for managing medications effectively.

Types of Diabetes Medications

There are several types of medications used to manage diabetes. The choice of medication depends on the type of diabetes, the severity of the condition, and individual health factors. These medications work in different ways to control blood sugar levels and may be used alone or in combination.

1. Oral Medications for Type 2 Diabetes

Oral medications are commonly prescribed for people with Type 2 diabetes to help control blood sugar. These medications work in various ways to increase insulin sensitivity, stimulate insulin production, or reduce glucose production by the liver.

- **Metformin**: The most commonly prescribed oral medication for Type 2 diabetes. It works by reducing glucose production in the liver and improving the body's response to insulin.
- **Sulfonylureas (e.g., glipizide, glyburide)**: These drugs stimulate the pancreas to release more insulin, helping lower blood sugar levels.
- **DPP-4 Inhibitors (e.g., sitagliptin, saxagliptin)**: These medications help increase insulin release and reduce glucose production by blocking an enzyme called DPP-4, which increases blood sugar.
- **SGLT-2 Inhibitors (e.g., empagliflozin, canagliflozin)**: These medications work by preventing the kidneys from reabsorbing glucose into the blood, leading to glucose being excreted in the urine.
- **Thiazolidinediones (e.g., pioglitazone, rosiglitazone)**: These medications improve insulin sensitivity, helping the body use insulin more effectively.
- **Meglitinides (e.g., repaglinide, nateglinide)**: These drugs help the pancreas produce more insulin in response to meals.

2. INSULIN THERAPY FOR TYPE 1 AND TYPE 2 DIABETES

Insulin is the main treatment for Type 1 diabetes, where the body does not produce insulin. It may also be prescribed for people with Type 2 diabetes when oral medications are no longer sufficient. Insulin therapy mimics the insulin the body would normally produce.

- **Types of Insulin**: Insulin comes in different forms based on how quickly it works and how long it lasts:
    - **Rapid-acting insulin**: Works quickly to reduce blood sugar after meals (e.g., insulin lispro, insulin aspart).
    - **Short-acting insulin**: Takes a bit longer to start working (e.g., regular insulin).
    - **Intermediate-acting insulin**: Works over a longer period (e.g., NPH insulin).
    - **Long-acting insulin**: Provides a steady release of insulin throughout the day and night (e.g., insulin glargine, insulin detemir).
- **Insulin Delivery**: Insulin can be delivered through injections or insulin pumps. Most people with Type 1 diabetes and some people with Type 2 diabetes may use multiple injections per day to maintain good blood sugar control.

3. Non-Insulin Injectable Medications

For people with Type 2 diabetes, non-insulin injectables may be prescribed to help lower blood sugar levels. These medications work by stimulating insulin production, reducing glucose production by the liver, or helping the body respond better to insulin.

- **GLP-1 Receptor Agonists (e.g., liraglutide, exenatide)**: These medications mimic a hormone called GLP-1 that helps regulate blood sugar by stimulating insulin release after meals and slowing down stomach emptying to promote satiety.
- **Amylin Analog (e.g., pramlintide)**: This injectable medication works by slowing down gastric emptying and reducing glucose production by the liver, helping control blood sugar.

HOW MEDICATIONS WORK

Diabetes medications work in various ways, depending on their class and mechanism of action. Here's how the different types of medications function:

- **Insulin**: Insulin lowers blood sugar by facilitating the transport of glucose into cells, where it can be used for energy or stored for later use.
- **Metformin**: It works by decreasing the liver's production of glucose and increasing the body's sensitivity to insulin.
- **Sulfonylureas**: They stimulate the pancreas to release more insulin, which helps lower blood sugar levels.

- **DPP-4 Inhibitors**: These medications inhibit the DPP-4 enzyme, which helps the body produce more insulin after meals and reduces the production of glucose from the liver.
- **SGLT-2 Inhibitors**: They prevent the kidneys from reabsorbing glucose, causing excess glucose to be excreted in the urine, which lowers blood sugar levels.
- **Thiazolidinediones**: These medications improve the body's ability to use insulin by increasing insulin sensitivity.
- **GLP-1 Agonists**: By mimicking the GLP-1 hormone, these drugs stimulate insulin release, reduce glucagon production (which raises blood sugar), and delay gastric emptying, leading to lower blood sugar levels.

Each class of medication has a specific role in managing blood sugar, and a healthcare provider may use a combination of these medications to tailor a treatment plan that works best for the individual.

Insulin Therapy

For those who need insulin therapy, understanding how to manage and administer insulin is crucial for effective blood sugar control.

Types of Insulin

- **Rapid-acting insulin**: Begins working within minutes and peaks in about 1 hour. It's typically used before meals to control blood sugar spikes.
- **Short-acting insulin**: Takes about 30 minutes to start working and peaks in about 2-3 hours. It is often used for meal-related blood sugar control.
- **Intermediate-acting insulin**: Works more gradually and is effective for up to 12 hours, often used for background or basal insulin coverage.
- **Long-acting insulin**: Provides a steady release of insulin over 24 hours, helping maintain stable blood sugar levels throughout the day and night.

INJECTION TECHNIQUES

- **Insulin Injections**: Insulin is usually injected subcutaneously (under the skin) using insulin pens or syringes. It's important to rotate injection sites to avoid tissue damage.
- **Insulin Pumps**: An insulin pump is a small device that delivers a continuous supply of insulin through a catheter placed under the skin. This method provides more precise control over insulin delivery.

TIMING OF INSULIN

- **Basal Insulin**: Long-acting or intermediate-acting insulin is taken once or twice a day to manage blood sugar between meals and overnight.
- **Bolus Insulin**: Rapid-acting or short-acting insulin is taken before meals to manage the rise in blood sugar that occurs after eating.

It's important to monitor blood sugar regularly and adjust insulin doses based on meals, physical activity, and other factors. Your healthcare provider will help you determine the right insulin regimen and timing for your needs.

MANAGING MEDICATIONS EFFECTIVELY

Effectively managing your medications is a key part of diabetes management. Here are strategies to help ensure that you take your medications as prescribed and deal with any challenges:

1. MEDICATION ADHERENCE

- **Create a Routine**: Take your medications at the same time every day to make them a part of your daily routine.
- **Use Reminders**: Set alarms on your phone or use medication reminder apps to help you remember when it's time to take your medications.
- **Track Your Medications**: Keep a log of your medications, doses, and any side effects to discuss with your healthcare provider during follow-up visits.

2. DEALING WITH SIDE EFFECTS

- Some medications may have side effects, such as nausea, weight gain, or low blood sugar (hypoglycemia). If you experience side effects, speak with your healthcare provider to explore alternative medications or strategies to manage them.

- **Hypoglycemia (Low Blood Sugar)**: If you're taking insulin or certain oral medications, you may experience hypoglycemia. Always carry a fast-acting source of sugar (e.g., glucose tablets, juice) and know the symptoms of low blood sugar.

3. ADJUSTING DOSES

- Your medication needs may change over time based on your blood sugar levels, lifestyle changes, or other health factors. Regular check-ins with your healthcare provider are important to ensure that your treatment plan is still effective.
- **Monitoring Blood Sugar**: Regular blood sugar monitoring helps you and your healthcare provider make adjustments to your medication regimen.

CONCLUSION

Medications are an essential part of diabetes management, helping to regulate blood sugar levels and reduce the risk of complications. Whether you're taking oral medications, insulin, or non-insulin injectables, it's important to understand how your medications work, the potential side effects, and how to manage them effectively. Working closely with your healthcare provider will help ensure that your medication regimen is tailored to your needs and helps you maintain optimal blood sugar control. In the next chapter, we will discuss the importance of monitoring blood sugar levels and how to do it effectively.

Chapter 8: Monitoring Blood Sugar Levels

Effective diabetes management requires regular monitoring of blood sugar levels. By tracking blood glucose levels, individuals with diabetes can understand how their body is responding to food, exercise, medications, and other factors. Monitoring not only helps to keep blood sugar levels within a healthy range, but it also enables you to make informed decisions about your treatment plan. This chapter explores why monitoring blood sugar is essential, the various tools available for monitoring, how to interpret your results, and advanced techniques for more detailed analysis.

Why Monitoring is Important

Monitoring blood sugar levels regularly is vital for several reasons:

1. **Tracking Blood Sugar Patterns**: Regular monitoring helps identify patterns in blood sugar levels throughout the day. Understanding how blood glucose responds to different foods, activities, medications, and stress is key to effective diabetes management. For example, you might notice that your blood sugar spikes after eating certain types of carbohydrates or that it drops after a workout.

2. **Adjusting Treatment Plans**: Monitoring provides feedback that helps you and your healthcare provider make adjustments to your

medication, diet, or lifestyle. If you notice consistently high or low blood sugar readings, your treatment plan may need to be adjusted.

3. **Preventing Complications**: Consistently well-managed blood sugar levels can prevent or delay the development of diabetes-related complications, such as heart disease, kidney problems, nerve damage, and vision issues.

4. **Understanding the Effectiveness of Treatment**: Regular monitoring helps you understand whether your treatment plan is working. If blood sugar levels are consistently outside of your target range, you may need to adjust your insulin dosage or other medications.

5. **Empowerment and Self-Management**: Frequent blood sugar checks help you take control of your diabetes. By knowing how different factors affect your blood glucose levels, you can make more informed decisions and improve your overall health.

How to Monitor Blood Sugar

There are several ways to monitor blood sugar levels, each with its own advantages and considerations. The most common methods include using a glucose meter, continuous glucose monitors (CGMs), and keeping a blood sugar log.

1. Glucose Meters

A glucose meter, also known as a glucometer, is a portable device that measures the amount of glucose in a blood sample. It is the most commonly used tool for blood sugar monitoring.

- **How it Works**: To use a glucose meter, you will need to prick your finger with a lancet (a small needle) to obtain a drop of blood. This blood drop is then placed on a test strip that is inserted into the glucose meter. The device will display your blood glucose level on the screen.
- **When to Test**: It's important to test at different times throughout the day, including:
    - **Fasting** (before breakfast)
    - **Pre- and post-meal** (1-2 hours after eating)
    - **Before bedtime**
    - **During periods of illness or stress**
- **Pros**: Affordable, portable, and widely available. It gives you a snapshot of your blood sugar at specific times.
- **Cons**: Requires finger pricks, which can be uncomfortable. You must remember to carry the meter and test strips.

2. CONTINUOUS GLUCOSE MONITORS (CGMs)

A continuous glucose monitor (CGM) is a device that continuously tracks glucose levels throughout the day and night.

- **How it Works**: A small sensor is inserted just under the skin, usually on the abdomen or arm. The sensor measures glucose levels in the interstitial fluid (the fluid between cells) and sends the data to a receiver or smartphone app. CGMs provide real-time data on your glucose levels, allowing for constant monitoring without needing finger pricks.

- **When to Test**: With a CGM, you don't need to manually test blood sugar as often, as it provides continuous data throughout the day. Some devices allow you to check your glucose levels in real-time or with a glance at your phone.

- **Pros**: Real-time data helps you spot trends and take immediate action if blood glucose levels are too high or too low. It provides more information than a glucose meter and reduces the need for frequent finger pricks.

- **Cons**: CGMs can be expensive, and sensors need to be replaced every few days to a week. They can also be less accurate than blood glucose meters under certain conditions.

3. KEEPING A BLOOD SUGAR LOG

Maintaining a blood sugar log is a simple and effective way to track your glucose levels over time. You can record the results from your glucose meter or CGM, along with other important details like the time of day, what you ate, how you were feeling, and any exercise or stress levels.

- **Why It's Important**: Keeping a log helps you and your healthcare team identify patterns, triggers, and potential issues with your diabetes management. It also helps your doctor determine if your current treatment plan is working effectively.
- **How to Keep a Log**: You can use a traditional paper log, a digital spreadsheet, or a smartphone app to track your results. Many apps are available that automatically sync with glucose meters or CGMs, making tracking easy.

INTERPRETING YOUR RESULTS

Understanding your blood sugar readings is crucial for effective diabetes management. Blood sugar levels fluctuate throughout the day and can be influenced by several factors, including food, physical activity, stress, illness, and medication. Here's what you should know about interpreting your results:

1. WHAT YOUR READINGS MEAN

Blood sugar targets vary depending on whether you have Type 1 or Type 2 diabetes, your age, and other individual factors. However, the general target ranges for a healthy blood sugar level are as follows:

- **Fasting (before meals)**: 80-130 mg/dL
- **Post-meal (1-2 hours after eating)**: Less than 180 mg/dL

- **Before bedtime**: 100-140 mg/dL

Note: Your healthcare provider will help you determine specific target ranges based on your health needs.

2. WHEN TO TAKE ACTION

- **High Blood Sugar (Hyperglycemia)**: Blood sugar levels higher than 180 mg/dL after meals or consistently above your target range may indicate hyperglycemia. High blood sugar can cause symptoms like increased thirst, frequent urination, fatigue, and blurred vision. If your blood sugar is consistently high, consult your healthcare provider to adjust your treatment plan.
- **Low Blood Sugar (Hypoglycemia)**: If your blood sugar drops below 70 mg/dL, it's considered hypoglycemia. Symptoms include shakiness, sweating, confusion, dizziness, and hunger. If you experience low blood sugar, take fast-acting carbohydrates like glucose tablets, juice, or regular soda to raise your blood sugar quickly.
- **Trend Monitoring**: Rather than focusing on individual readings, monitoring trends over time is crucial. Consistent high or low readings over several days or weeks may indicate that adjustments need to be made to your medication, diet, or exercise routine.

In addition to regular blood sugar testing, there are other advanced monitoring techniques that can help provide more detailed insights into your diabetes management.

1. KETONE TESTING

Ketone testing is essential for people with Type 1 diabetes, particularly if blood sugar levels are consistently high. Ketones are produced when the body starts breaking down fat for energy due to insufficient insulin, a condition known as diabetic ketoacidosis (DKA), which can be life-threatening.

- **How to Test for Ketones**: Ketones can be detected through urine tests or blood tests. If your blood sugar is over 240 mg/dL and you're feeling unwell, check for ketones. High ketone levels may require medical intervention.

2. A1C MONITORING

The A1C test measures the average blood glucose level over the past 2-3 months. It is an essential tool for long-term blood sugar management and provides a snapshot of how well your diabetes is controlled over time.

- **Target A1C Levels**: The general target for most people with diabetes is an A1C below 7%. However, your healthcare provider may recommend a different target based on your specific health needs.
- **Frequency of Testing**: The A1C test is typically done every 3-6 months. It's an important marker for assessing your overall diabetes management.

3. Continuous Glucose Monitoring (CGM) Data Integration

Some CGM systems provide reports that offer deep insights into blood glucose trends, including graphs and charts that show how blood sugar changes over the course of a day. These reports can help you and your healthcare team make more precise adjustments to your treatment plan.

Conclusion

Regularly monitoring your blood sugar levels is a cornerstone of effective diabetes management. Whether you use a traditional glucose meter, a continuous glucose monitor, or both, tracking your blood sugar levels helps you make informed decisions about your diet, exercise, and medications. By interpreting your results, understanding trends, and utilizing advanced monitoring techniques, you can take control of your diabetes and reduce the risk of complications. The next chapter will focus on managing stress and emotional well-being, which also plays a significant role in diabetes control.

Section 3:

Living Well with Diabetes

Chapter 9: Managing Stress and Emotional Well-being

Living with diabetes requires not only managing physical health but also taking care of your emotional well-being. Stress can have a significant impact on blood sugar levels, and chronic stress can make diabetes management more challenging. This chapter explores the connection between stress and blood sugar, various stress management techniques, and how to cope with diabetes-related stress. It also emphasizes the importance of building a support system to help manage the emotional aspects of living with diabetes.

The Connection Between Stress and Blood Sugar

Stress, both physical and emotional, can affect blood sugar levels in a variety of ways. When you experience stress, your body activates the "fight-or-flight" response, releasing stress hormones like cortisol and adrenaline. These hormones prepare your body to deal with perceived threats, but they can also cause blood sugar levels to rise.

- **Cortisol and Blood Sugar:** Cortisol, the body's primary stress hormone, can increase glucose production in the liver and reduce the body's sensitivity to insulin. This means that during times of stress, your body may produce more glucose, while insulin becomes less effective at moving that glucose into your cells. This can lead to higher blood sugar levels, which are particularly concerning for people with diabetes.

- **Adrenaline's Impact**: Adrenaline (also known as epinephrine) is another hormone released during stress. It prepares your body for quick action by increasing heart rate and blood sugar levels. While this response is helpful in the short term, prolonged stress can make it harder to manage blood sugar effectively.
- **Chronic Stress**: Chronic stress can lead to a cycle where elevated blood sugar levels worsen, which in turn can lead to more stress about managing diabetes. This can create a vicious cycle, making stress management an essential part of diabetes care.

STRESS MANAGEMENT TECHNIQUES

Since stress is unavoidable in life, learning how to manage it is a key component of living well with diabetes. The following techniques can help reduce the impact of stress on your blood sugar levels and improve your overall emotional well-being:

1. MEDITATION

Meditation involves focusing your mind and calming your body to reduce stress. Mindfulness meditation, in particular, has been shown to be effective in lowering stress and improving blood sugar control in people with diabetes. Regular practice can help you feel more grounded and better equipped to handle stress.

- **How to Practice**: Find a quiet space, close your eyes, and focus on your breath. You can use guided meditation apps or simply focus on the present moment without judgment. Aim for 10-20 minutes of practice daily.

2. DEEP BREATHING

Deep breathing exercises are simple yet effective techniques for reducing stress. When you breathe deeply, you activate the body's relaxation response, which helps counter the effects of stress hormones.

- **How to Practice**: Sit or lie down in a comfortable position. Inhale slowly through your nose, allowing your abdomen to rise as you fill your lungs with air. Exhale slowly through your mouth, releasing tension. Repeat for 5-10 minutes.

3. YOGA

Yoga combines physical postures, controlled breathing, and meditation to reduce stress and promote relaxation. It has been shown to lower blood sugar levels and improve insulin sensitivity, making it especially beneficial for individuals with diabetes.

- **How to Practice**: You don't need to be an expert to benefit from yoga. Begin with basic poses like child's pose, downward dog, and gentle stretching. Many yoga classes or apps offer beginner-friendly sessions.

4. PROGRESSIVE MUSCLE RELAXATION (PMR)

Progressive muscle relaxation involves tensing and then relaxing different muscle groups in the body. This technique helps release physical tension and promotes a sense of calm.

- **How to Practice**: Starting from your feet, work your way up through the body, tensing each muscle group for 5-10 seconds, then relaxing it for 20-30 seconds. Focus on the sensations of tension and release.

5. MINDFUL MOVEMENT

Engaging in mindful movement activities, such as walking, tai chi, or swimming, can also reduce stress. The key is to focus on your body's movements, the rhythm of your breath, and the sensations you experience during the activity.

- **How to Practice**: Choose an activity you enjoy and focus on the sensation of movement. Notice how your body feels as it moves through space and try to quiet your mind.

Living with a chronic condition like diabetes can be emotionally taxing. It's not uncommon for individuals to experience feelings of frustration, anxiety, or depression as they navigate the challenges of managing their health. Learning how to cope with these emotions is vital for maintaining both physical and emotional well-being.

1. ACKNOWLEDGE YOUR FEELINGS

It's important to acknowledge the emotional toll that diabetes can have on your life. Whether you feel overwhelmed by the constant need for monitoring, frustrated by fluctuating blood sugar levels, or sad about lifestyle changes, it's normal to have these emotions. Recognizing and validating your feelings is the first step toward healing.

2. PRACTICE SELF-COMPASSION

Managing diabetes can be difficult, and it's easy to be hard on yourself when things don't go as planned. However, practicing self-compassion—treating yourself with kindness and understanding—is essential for your emotional well-being. Recognize that setbacks are part of the journey and be gentle with yourself when things don't go perfectly.

3. Seek Professional Support

If you are feeling particularly overwhelmed, anxious, or depressed, consider seeking help from a mental health professional. Cognitive-behavioral therapy (CBT), counseling, or support groups can provide valuable tools for managing emotional distress and improving your overall outlook on living with diabetes.

- **Therapy**: Talking to a psychologist or therapist can help you address underlying emotional concerns, learn coping strategies, and develop a positive mindset.
- **Support Groups**: Joining a diabetes support group can provide a sense of community and understanding. Sharing experiences with others facing similar challenges can offer emotional relief and helpful insights into managing diabetes.

Building a Support System

Living with diabetes doesn't have to be a solitary journey. Having a strong support system can make all the difference in how you manage your condition and maintain your emotional well-being.

1. Family and Friends

Having a strong network of family and friends can provide emotional support and encouragement. They can help you stick to your treatment plan, join you in healthy activities, and offer understanding when you're feeling frustrated or stressed. Don't be afraid to share your struggles with those you trust—they may not always have the answers, but they can offer a listening ear.

2. DIABETES EDUCATORS

Diabetes educators are healthcare professionals who specialize in helping individuals with diabetes manage their condition. They can provide valuable information about blood sugar control, medications, meal planning, and emotional support.

3. ONLINE AND IN-PERSON SUPPORT GROUPS

Support groups for people with diabetes are available both online and in person. These groups can help you connect with others who understand your challenges, share tips, and provide moral support. Whether in-person or through online forums, the sense of community can be invaluable.

4. HEALTHCARE PROVIDERS

Your healthcare team, including your endocrinologist, dietitian, and primary care physician, plays an essential role in supporting your diabetes management. They can help you stay on track with your treatment plan and provide guidance on managing stress and emotional well-being.

CONCLUSION

Managing diabetes is not just about controlling blood sugar levels; it's about taking care of your mental and emotional health as well. By understanding the connection between stress and blood sugar, implementing stress management techniques, and seeking emotional support, you can live a balanced and fulfilling life with diabetes. In the next chapter, we'll explore how to make long-term lifestyle changes that support diabetes management, including developing healthy habits that will serve you for life.

Chapter 10: Sleep and Diabetes

Good sleep is crucial for maintaining overall health, but its significance is especially apparent when it comes to managing diabetes. Sleep affects many aspects of physical health, including insulin sensitivity, hormone regulation, and blood sugar control. Unfortunately, individuals with diabetes often face sleep disturbances that can worsen blood sugar management. In this chapter, we'll explore how sleep influences diabetes, provide tips for improving sleep quality, and discuss the relationship between sleep apnea and diabetes.

The Role of Sleep in Blood Sugar Control

Sleep and blood sugar levels are closely connected. When you sleep, your body undergoes various processes that influence how your body uses and stores glucose. Here's how sleep can impact diabetes management:

1. Insulin Sensitivity

During sleep, the body's insulin sensitivity typically improves. Insulin is the hormone that helps regulate blood sugar by moving glucose from the blood into cells. Lack of sleep, however, can decrease insulin sensitivity, making it harder for your body to use insulin effectively. This can result in higher blood sugar levels, which can complicate diabetes management.

- **Studies on Sleep and Insulin Sensitivity**: Research has shown that poor or insufficient sleep can increase insulin resistance, especially in individuals with Type 2 diabetes. Over time, this can contribute to higher fasting blood sugar levels and make it more challenging to control diabetes.

2. HORMONAL REGULATION

Sleep also plays a significant role in the regulation of key hormones that affect blood sugar levels. One of the most important hormones related to blood sugar is cortisol, a stress hormone that is typically higher in the morning to help you wake up. However, when sleep is disrupted, cortisol levels can become elevated throughout the night and day, leading to higher blood sugar levels. Additionally, insufficient sleep can lead to an increase in hunger hormones (ghrelin) and a decrease in hormones that signal satiety (leptin), which can lead to overeating and further complications in managing blood sugar.

3. BLOOD SUGAR FLUCTUATIONS

Sleep disturbances, such as insomnia or frequent waking, can lead to fluctuations in blood sugar levels. This is particularly true for individuals with diabetes who may experience "dawn phenomenon" (higher blood sugar levels in the morning) or "nocturnal hypoglycemia" (low blood sugar during sleep), both of which are influenced by sleep patterns.

Improving sleep quality is essential for managing blood sugar levels and enhancing overall health. Here are several tips to help you get better sleep and ensure that your body is properly rested and regulated:

1. MAINTAIN A CONSISTENT SLEEP SCHEDULE

Going to bed and waking up at the same time every day helps regulate your body's internal clock. Consistency reinforces your natural circadian rhythm, making it easier to fall asleep and wake up feeling refreshed.

- **Tip**: Set a bedtime routine to wind down—this can include activities like reading, listening to calming music, or practicing relaxation exercises before bed.

2. CREATE A SLEEP-FRIENDLY ENVIRONMENT

A sleep-friendly environment is dark, quiet, and cool. If possible, eliminate noise, reduce light exposure (especially from electronic devices), and ensure that your bedroom temperature is comfortable for sleep (usually between 60–67°F or 15-19°C).

- **TIP:** Consider blackout curtains, white noise machines, or earplugs to block out distractions. Avoid using screens (phone, computer, TV) at least 30 minutes to an hour before bedtime, as blue light can interfere with melatonin production.

3. EXERCISE REGULARLY

Regular physical activity can improve both the quality and duration of sleep. Exercise helps reduce stress, improves mood, and promotes relaxation—all of which are beneficial for sleep.

- **TIP:** Aim to finish vigorous exercise at least 3 hours before bedtime, as exercising too close to sleep may have the opposite effect by increasing energy and making it harder to fall asleep.

4. LIMIT CAFFEINE AND ALCOHOL INTAKE

Both caffeine and alcohol can interfere with your ability to fall asleep and achieve deep, restorative sleep. Caffeine, a stimulant, can keep you awake for hours, while alcohol can disrupt the later stages of the sleep cycle.

- **Tip:** Limit caffeine intake after the afternoon and avoid alcohol close to bedtime to ensure it doesn't interfere with your sleep quality.

5. PRACTICE RELAXATION TECHNIQUES

Stress and anxiety can prevent restful sleep, so incorporating relaxation techniques before bed can be helpful. Mindfulness meditation, progressive muscle relaxation, deep breathing exercises, and yoga can all promote relaxation and ease stress.

- TIP: Try deep breathing exercises, where you inhale slowly for 4 seconds, hold for 7 seconds, and exhale for 8 seconds. This can activate the body's parasympathetic nervous system, helping you feel more relaxed.

MANAGING SLEEP APNEA

Sleep apnea, a condition where breathing repeatedly stops and starts during sleep, is more common in people with diabetes, particularly those with Type 2 diabetes. Sleep apnea can lead to fragmented sleep, low oxygen levels, and increased stress on the heart and blood vessels, further complicating blood sugar management.

1. WHAT IS SLEEP APNEA?

Sleep apnea is a sleep disorder characterized by repeated interruptions in breathing during sleep. The most common type is obstructive sleep apnea (OSA), where the muscles in the throat relax too much and block the airway. This can lead to frequent awakenings throughout the night and decreased oxygen levels in the blood, which in turn affects heart function and blood sugar regulation.

- **Symptoms of Sleep Apnea**: Loud snoring, choking or gasping during sleep, excessive daytime fatigue, difficulty concentrating, and morning headaches.

2. THE LINK BETWEEN DIABETES AND SLEEP APNEA

Research suggests that untreated sleep apnea can contribute to poor blood sugar control in individuals with diabetes. People with sleep apnea experience intermittent oxygen deprivation, which can lead to insulin resistance, a common issue in Type 2 diabetes. Additionally, poor sleep quality from sleep apnea can increase levels of stress hormones like cortisol, which further affects blood sugar regulation.

3. TREATMENT OPTIONS FOR SLEEP APNEA

The most effective treatment for sleep apnea is the use of a Continuous Positive Airway Pressure (CPAP) machine. This device delivers a steady flow of air to keep the airways open during sleep.

- **CPAP Therapy**: A CPAP machine can help reduce the frequency of apneas (breathing stoppages) and improve overall sleep quality. When used consistently, CPAP therapy can help improve blood sugar control in people with diabetes.

- **Lifestyle Modifications**: In addition to CPAP therapy, lifestyle changes like weight loss, sleeping on your side, and avoiding alcohol or sedatives before bed can help reduce the severity of sleep apnea.

4. REGULAR MONITORING AND CONSULTATION

If you suspect you have sleep apnea, it's essential to consult with a healthcare provider for diagnosis and treatment. A sleep study (polysomnography) is typically performed to confirm the condition and determine the severity of apnea episodes.

CONCLUSION

Sleep is a vital component of diabetes management, influencing insulin sensitivity, hormone regulation, and overall blood sugar control. By making sleep a priority, you can help manage your diabetes more effectively. Improving sleep quality, managing conditions like sleep apnea, and establishing healthy sleep habits are essential steps toward better health and well-being. In the next chapter, we will explore how to maintain a balanced and sustainable lifestyle while living with diabetes.

Chapter 11: Avoiding Alcohol and Smoking

Living with diabetes requires making conscious decisions to protect your health. Two common habits—alcohol consumption and smoking—can significantly impact blood sugar levels, overall diabetes management, and the risk of complications. In this chapter, we'll explore how alcohol and smoking affect diabetes, provide strategies for safe alcohol consumption, and offer tips for quitting smoking.

The Effects of Alcohol on Diabetes

Alcohol can have both short-term and long-term effects on blood sugar levels, making it important for people with diabetes to understand how it interacts with their condition and their medications.

1. How Alcohol Impacts Blood Sugar Levels

- **Initial Sugar Spike:** When consumed, alcohol can cause a rapid increase in blood sugar, particularly in sugary mixed drinks or cocktails. However, alcohol alone—especially in higher quantities—can also lower blood sugar levels by interfering with the liver's ability to release glucose into the bloodstream.

- **Liver Function and Blood Sugar Control**: The liver is responsible for releasing glucose into the blood when levels are low. Alcohol can inhibit this process, which means your blood sugar may drop several hours after drinking, especially if you are on insulin or other blood-sugar-lowering medications. This can lead to hypoglycemia (low blood sugar), which can be dangerous if not addressed immediately.

- **Risk of Hypoglycemia**: Drinking alcohol without food can significantly increase the risk of hypoglycemia, particularly if you are using insulin or sulfonylureas. This is because alcohol impairs the liver's ability to release glucose and prolongs the effects of low blood sugar.

2. INTERACTIONS WITH MEDICATIONS

- **Medication Impact**: Alcohol can interact with various diabetes medications, making it harder to manage blood sugar effectively. For example, alcohol can increase the risk of side effects from medications like metformin, sulfonylureas, and insulin, and alter their effectiveness.

- **Hypoglycemia and Medications**: Insulin and other blood sugar-lowering drugs can cause hypoglycemia, and alcohol can intensify this risk. It's important to monitor your blood sugar closely if you plan to drink and adjust your medication accordingly with the guidance of your healthcare provider.

If you choose to consume alcohol, it's important to do so safely and in a way that minimizes the risks to your diabetes management. Here are some strategies:

1. Know Your Limits

Moderation is key. For individuals with diabetes, it's essential to limit alcohol intake to avoid fluctuations in blood sugar. The American Diabetes Association (ADA) recommends that women consume no more than one drink per day and men no more than two drinks per day.

- **What is one drink?**: One drink is defined as:
    - 12 ounces of beer (with 5% alcohol content)
    - 5 ounces of wine (with 12% alcohol content)
    - 1.5 ounces of distilled spirits (such as vodka, whiskey, or rum)

2. Never Drink on an Empty Stomach

Eating food while drinking can help stabilize your blood sugar and prevent alcohol-induced hypoglycemia. Always eat a balanced meal or snack that includes protein, fiber, and healthy fats before or while drinking.

- **Tip**: Avoid sugary or high-carbohydrate snacks, as these can cause spikes in blood sugar. Focus on foods that balance the alcohol's effects, such as nuts, cheese, or lean proteins.

3. MONITOR YOUR BLOOD SUGAR LEVELS

If you plan to drink, it's important to check your blood sugar levels before and after drinking. This will help you understand how your body reacts to alcohol and allow you to take action if your blood sugar drops too low.

- **Use a Continuous Glucose Monitor (CGM)**: If you have access to a CGM, it can provide real-time data on your blood sugar levels, helping you respond quickly to any changes that may occur while drinking.

4. BE AWARE OF HIDDEN SUGARS

Some alcoholic beverages, like sweet wines, flavored liquors, and mixed drinks, can contain high levels of sugar, which may cause your blood sugar to spike. Opt for drinks with fewer added sugars, such as straight spirits mixed with water, seltzer, or low-calorie mixers.

THE IMPACT OF SMOKING ON DIABETES

Smoking is a significant risk factor for a variety of health complications, and it can be particularly harmful to individuals with diabetes. Here's why:

1. Smoking Increases the Risk of Complications

- **Cardiovascular Disease**: Smokers are more likely to develop heart disease, which is already a higher risk for individuals with diabetes. Smoking accelerates the process of atherosclerosis (hardening of the arteries) and increases the risk of heart attacks, strokes, and peripheral artery disease.
- **Nerve Damage**: Smoking exacerbates the risk of diabetic neuropathy (nerve damage), as it can impair blood circulation and limit the delivery of oxygen and nutrients to nerve cells.
- **Kidney Disease**: Smoking also contributes to kidney damage in people with diabetes, as it can increase the risk of diabetic nephropathy (kidney disease), which may lead to kidney failure over time.
- **Eye Problems**: Smokers with diabetes are at an increased risk of diabetic retinopathy, a condition that can lead to vision loss and blindness. Smoking contributes to the damage of blood vessels in the eyes.

2. Smoking Affects Insulin Sensitivity

Smoking can worsen insulin resistance, a key factor in managing Type 2 diabetes. The chemicals in tobacco smoke interfere with the body's ability to respond to insulin effectively, making it harder to control blood sugar levels.

- **Increased Blood Sugar Levels**: Smoking may lead to higher blood sugar levels, which can make it more difficult to achieve target glucose levels, especially over time.

Tips for Quitting Smoking

Quitting smoking is one of the best decisions you can make for your health, especially if you have diabetes. Although it can be challenging, there are various strategies and resources that can support your journey:

1. Seek Professional Help

Consult with your healthcare provider about strategies and tools that can help you quit smoking. They may recommend nicotine replacement therapies (patches, gum, lozenges) or prescription medications like varenicline (Chantix) or bupropion (Zyban) to help manage cravings.

2. Create a Quit Plan

Set a quit date and prepare yourself by removing cigarettes, lighters, and ashtrays from your environment. Inform friends, family, and colleagues about your decision to quit so they can support you along the way.

- **Tip**: Identify triggers that make you want to smoke, such as stress or after meals, and find healthier alternatives to cope with these situations, like deep breathing or taking a walk.

3. USE SUPPORT NETWORKS

Support groups—either in-person or online—can provide motivation and encouragement during your quit journey. You can also reach out to a counselor or therapist for guidance on managing the emotional challenges of quitting smoking.

- **Online Resources**: Websites like Smokefree.gov and quit lines (such as 1-800-QUIT-NOW) offer free support and advice.

4. STAY ACTIVE AND ENGAGED

Physical activity can help distract you from cravings, reduce stress, and improve your mood. Regular exercise can also improve your insulin sensitivity, helping with diabetes management.

- **Tip**: Engage in activities you enjoy, such as walking, swimming, or yoga, to keep your mind off smoking.

5. Be Patient with Yourself

Quitting smoking is a process, and it's normal to face setbacks. If you slip up, don't be discouraged. Simply acknowledge the mistake, recommit to your goal, and keep moving forward.

Conclusion

Both alcohol and smoking can significantly affect diabetes management and increase the risk of complications. By understanding the impact of these habits on your health and taking proactive steps to minimize their effects, you can better manage your condition. If you choose to drink, do so in moderation and with caution, and consider quitting smoking for a healthier, more balanced life. Remember, every positive change you make contributes to better overall health and a stronger ability to manage your diabetes.

Chapter 12: Managing Diabetes in Special Situations

Living with diabetes means adapting to various life situations and challenges. From traveling to pregnancy, from managing diabetes at work to handling illness, each scenario requires careful planning and consideration. This chapter provides guidance on how to manage diabetes in special situations, ensuring you maintain control of your health no matter where life takes you.

Traveling with Diabetes

Traveling can be exciting, but it also requires special considerations for individuals with diabetes. Whether you're going on a short trip or an international adventure, here are the key things to keep in mind:

1. Preparing for Travel

- **Pack Supplies:** Ensure that you have enough diabetes supplies, including insulin, blood glucose meters, test strips, syringes or pens, and any other medications. It's always a good idea to pack extra in case of delays or emergencies. Keep these supplies in your carry-on bag, as they could be lost or damaged in checked luggage.

- **Prescription Documentation:** Carry a letter from your doctor that explains your diabetes diagnosis and your need for medication, especially if you're traveling internationally. This can help you avoid issues with airport security or customs.

- **Know Local Healthcare Options**: Before traveling, research the healthcare facilities available at your destination in case you need medical assistance. Keep a list of emergency contacts and know where the nearest hospital or doctor is located.

2. MANAGING TIME ZONES

- **Adjusting Insulin Timing**: If you're traveling across time zones, you may need to adjust the timing of your insulin injections or meals to maintain stable blood sugar levels. Speak with your healthcare provider before traveling to discuss how best to modify your routine.
- **Monitor Blood Sugar**: Traveling can disrupt your regular schedule, so it's important to check your blood sugar more frequently during the first few days in a new time zone to identify any changes and address them quickly.

3. HANDLING EMERGENCIES

- **Know What to Do in a Crisis**: In case of low or high blood sugar, have a plan in place. Carry fast-acting glucose for hypoglycemia (low blood sugar), such as glucose tablets, juice, or candy. For hyperglycemia (high blood sugar), have your insulin or prescribed medication handy and take it according to your doctor's recommendations.

- **Emergency Contact Information**: Write down your doctor's contact information, the address and phone number of your accommodation, and the contact information for any local diabetes organizations in case you need help while traveling.

DIABETES AND WORK

Managing diabetes at work can present challenges, especially when balancing your blood sugar, workload, and stress. Here are some strategies to help you succeed in the workplace while keeping your diabetes in check:

1. MANAGING DIABETES AT WORK

- **Schedule Regular Breaks**: Taking short breaks throughout the day to check your blood sugar, eat healthy snacks, and stretch can help prevent blood sugar fluctuations. Ensure that you have time to take medications or insulin as needed.
- **Bring Healthy Snacks**: Pack a variety of healthy snacks that can help stabilize your blood sugar levels, such as nuts, fruit, yogurt, or whole-grain crackers. Avoid high-sugar or processed snacks, as they can cause rapid blood sugar spikes.

- **Hydrate**: Staying hydrated is essential for managing diabetes, so make sure to drink plenty of water throughout the day. Avoid sugary drinks, as they can affect your blood sugar.

2. DEALING WITH STRESS AT WORK

- **Stress and Blood Sugar**: Work-related stress can affect your blood sugar levels, either by raising it due to the release of stress hormones or lowering it if you skip meals or snacks. Finding effective ways to manage stress is essential for your overall diabetes control.
- **Stress Management Techniques**: Consider practicing mindfulness, deep breathing, or meditation during the workday to lower stress levels. Taking breaks to move around or stretch can also help alleviate physical tension and improve circulation.

3. KNOWING YOUR RIGHTS

- **Workplace Discrimination**: Under the Americans with Disabilities Act (ADA) and similar laws in many countries, people with diabetes are protected from discrimination in the workplace. This means that you are entitled to reasonable accommodations, such as the ability to take breaks for blood sugar monitoring, insulin injections, and eating meals or snacks.
- **Communicate with Your Employer**: If needed, have an open conversation with your employer about your diabetes management

requirements. You may need accommodations for flexible break times or a private space to manage your blood sugar.

PREGNANCY AND DIABETES

Pregnancy brings unique challenges for women with diabetes, whether you have pre-existing diabetes (Type 1 or Type 2) or develop gestational diabetes during pregnancy. Here's how to manage diabetes during pregnancy:

1. MANAGING PRE-EXISTING DIABETES DURING PREGNANCY

- **Consult Your Doctor**: If you have diabetes and are planning to become pregnant, it's important to have a preconception visit with your healthcare provider to optimize your blood sugar control before conceiving. Maintaining stable blood sugar levels early in pregnancy reduces the risk of complications for both you and the baby.
- **Frequent Blood Sugar Monitoring**: Throughout pregnancy, you will need to monitor your blood sugar levels more frequently, as pregnancy hormones can affect insulin sensitivity. Your doctor may adjust your insulin doses or medication as needed to keep blood sugar levels within a healthy range.
- **Healthy Diet and Exercise**: Eating a balanced diet and staying active during pregnancy can help control blood sugar and promote a healthy

pregnancy. Work with your healthcare team to create a plan that meets the needs of both you and your baby.

2. GESTATIONAL DIABETES

- **What is Gestational Diabetes?** Gestational diabetes is a type of diabetes that occurs during pregnancy and typically resolves after childbirth. However, it can increase the risk of developing Type 2 diabetes later in life. Managing blood sugar levels during pregnancy is crucial for both maternal and fetal health.

- **Monitoring and Treatment:** Women with gestational diabetes often need to monitor blood sugar levels regularly. Treatment may include changes to diet, exercise, and, in some cases, insulin or oral medication. Your healthcare provider will help guide you in managing gestational diabetes to ensure a healthy pregnancy.

3. POSTPARTUM CARE

- **Postpartum Blood Sugar Monitoring:** After childbirth, it's important to continue monitoring your blood sugar levels to ensure that gestational diabetes has resolved. You will likely be tested for Type 2 diabetes six to 12 weeks after delivery, especially if you had gestational diabetes.

- **Breastfeeding:** Breastfeeding has several benefits, including helping to regulate blood sugar levels for both mother and baby. Work with your healthcare provider to create a postpartum plan for managing your diabetes and maintaining a healthy lifestyle.

DEALING WITH ILLNESS AND SICK DAYS

When you're sick, your diabetes management plan may need to be adjusted. Illness, whether it's a cold, flu, or infection, can affect blood sugar levels in different ways. Here's how to handle diabetes when you're not feeling well:

1. ILLNESS AND BLOOD SUGAR CONTROL

- **Blood Sugar Fluctuations**: Illness can cause blood sugar levels to rise due to the stress response and the release of stress hormones like cortisol. Alternatively, if you have a decreased appetite or difficulty eating, blood sugar may drop. This makes it important to monitor your blood sugar more frequently when you're sick.
- **Adjusting Medication**: When you're sick, your insulin needs may change. Work with your healthcare provider to adjust your insulin doses or medications as needed. In some cases, you may need to use extra insulin to manage higher blood sugar levels.

2. STAYING HYDRATED AND EATING WELL

- **Hydration is Key**: Dehydration can worsen blood sugar control. Drink plenty of fluids, such as water, broth, and sugar-free drinks, to stay hydrated and help flush out excess sugar from your system.

- **Eat Small, Balanced Meals**: If you're not feeling hungry, try eating small meals or snacks throughout the day to maintain blood sugar control. Foods that are easy to digest, such as soup, toast, or crackers, can help you maintain energy and stabilize blood sugar levels.

3. SEEK MEDICAL HELP IF NEEDED

- **When to Call Your Doctor**: If your blood sugar levels remain consistently high or low, or if you're unable to manage your blood sugar during illness, contact your healthcare provider. Illness can sometimes cause complications that require medical attention, especially if you're unable to keep food or liquids down.

CONCLUSION

Managing diabetes during special situations, such as traveling, pregnancy, work, or illness, requires extra attention and preparation. By staying informed and proactive, you can maintain stable blood sugar levels and handle any challenges that come your way. Remember, with the right support and strategies, you can successfully navigate these situations and continue to live well with diabetes.

SECTION 4

ADVANCED DIABETES MANAGEMENT

Chapter 13: Preventing Complications

Diabetes can lead to a variety of complications if not managed properly. However, with proactive care and regular monitoring, many of these complications can be prevented or delayed. This chapter focuses on the most common complications associated with diabetes, how to detect them early, and steps to take to minimize the risks. We will also discuss the importance of foot care and oral health, both of which are often overlooked but crucial for maintaining overall health in individuals with diabetes.

---

1. Common Complications of Diabetes

Diabetes, if not controlled effectively, can affect multiple organs and systems in the body. Understanding the most common complications can help you take preventive actions and manage your health effectively.

1.1 Heart Disease

- **Increased Risk:** People with diabetes are at a higher risk of developing heart disease and related conditions like high blood pressure, high cholesterol, and stroke. High blood sugar levels can damage blood vessels and nerves that control the heart, leading to cardiovascular complications.

- **Prevention**: Managing your blood sugar, maintaining a healthy weight, eating a balanced diet low in unhealthy fats and salt, and exercising regularly can significantly reduce the risk of heart disease. Regular monitoring of cholesterol and blood pressure levels is also essential.

1.2 Neuropathy (Nerve Damage)

- **Types of Neuropathy**: Diabetic neuropathy can affect various parts of the body, including the feet, legs, hands, and arms. It occurs when high blood sugar levels damage the nerves over time, leading to symptoms such as tingling, numbness, pain, and even loss of sensation.
- **Prevention**: Tight blood sugar control is essential in preventing or slowing the progression of neuropathy. Regular foot inspections, wearing comfortable shoes, and managing blood sugar effectively can help prevent nerve damage.

1.3 Kidney Disease (Diabetic Nephropathy)

- **Impact on Kidneys**: High blood sugar levels can damage the small blood vessels in the kidneys, impairing their ability to filter waste and excess fluids from the body. Over time, this can lead to kidney failure, a serious and life-threatening condition.
- **Prevention**: Regular kidney function tests (such as albumin-to-creatinine ratio), controlling blood pressure, and maintaining good blood sugar levels are critical for preventing kidney disease. Adequate

hydration and avoiding excess use of over-the-counter medications (like NSAIDs) can also protect kidney health.

- **Diabetic Retinopathy**: Diabetes can damage the blood vessels in the retina, leading to vision problems and even blindness. This condition often develops slowly and may not show symptoms in the early stages.
- **Prevention**: Regular eye exams are essential for early detection of diabetic retinopathy. Keeping blood sugar levels under control, managing blood pressure, and avoiding smoking can help prevent damage to the eyes.

---

2. Early Detection and Management

Preventing complications relies heavily on early detection and proactive management. Here are some key strategies for managing your health and detecting problems early:

- **Eye Exams**: Schedule a comprehensive eye exam at least once a year. Early detection of diabetic retinopathy can lead to treatments that help prevent significant vision loss.

- **Kidney Function Tests**: Get regular tests to check for early signs of kidney damage, such as the albumin-to-creatinine ratio. Early intervention can prevent or delay the progression of kidney disease.

- **Foot Exams**: Have a thorough foot examination at least once a year to look for signs of nerve damage, poor circulation, and infection.

- **Cholesterol and Blood Pressure Monitoring**: Regularly monitor your cholesterol and blood pressure levels to assess cardiovascular risk. Keeping both within a healthy range is crucial for preventing heart disease.

2.2 RECOGNIZING SYMPTOMS EARLY

Being aware of early symptoms of complications can help you take action before they become severe. Some common signs of complications include:

- **Heart Disease**: Chest pain, shortness of breath, or swelling in the legs can be signs of heart problems.

- **Neuropathy**: Tingling, numbness, or a burning sensation in the hands or feet could indicate nerve damage.

- **Kidney Disease**: Swelling in the feet or ankles, fatigue, and changes in urination may suggest kidney problems.

- **Eye Problems**: Blurry vision, floaters, or difficulty seeing in low light could indicate diabetic retinopathy.

If you notice any of these symptoms, consult your healthcare provider immediately for further testing and treatment.

---

3. Foot Care

Foot problems are one of the most common complications of diabetes, yet they are often preventable with proper care. Nerve damage and poor circulation in the feet increase the risk of injury, infection, and even amputation. Proper foot care is essential for those with diabetes.

3.1 PREVENTING FOOT COMPLICATIONS

- **Daily Foot Inspections:** Check your feet every day for cuts, blisters, redness, swelling, or signs of infection. Pay close attention to areas between your toes and the soles of your feet.
- **Keep Feet Clean and Dry:** Wash your feet daily with lukewarm water and mild soap. Dry them thoroughly, especially between the toes, to prevent fungal infections.
- **Wear Proper Footwear:** Choose shoes that fit well and avoid tight, restrictive shoes that can cause blisters or pressure sores. Avoid walking barefoot, as this increases the risk of injury.
- **Trim Toenails Carefully:** Cut your toenails straight across and avoid cutting them too short to prevent ingrown nails.

- **Podiatrist Visits**: If you have foot problems or are at high risk of complications, schedule regular visits to a podiatrist (foot specialist). They can assess the condition of your feet, offer preventive care, and provide treatments for any existing foot issues.

---

4. Oral Health

Oral health is an often-overlooked aspect of diabetes management. Diabetes increases the risk of gum disease (periodontal disease), which can, in turn, make it more difficult to control blood sugar. High blood sugar levels contribute to dry mouth, which increases the risk of cavities and gum infections.

4.1 THE LINK BETWEEN DIABETES AND GUM DISEASE

- **How Diabetes Affects Oral Health**: High blood sugar levels can lead to dry mouth, reduced saliva, and an increase in plaque buildup, all of which contribute to gum disease. Gum disease, in turn, can cause further elevation of blood sugar levels and lead to complications in diabetes management.

- **Signs of Gum Disease**: Symptoms include swollen, bleeding gums, bad breath, loose teeth, or painful chewing. If left untreated, gum disease can lead to tooth loss and infections that affect overall health.

4.2 MAINTAINING ORAL HEALTH

- **Brush and Floss Regularly**: Brush your teeth at least twice a day with fluoride toothpaste, and floss daily to remove food particles and plaque from between your teeth.
- **Regular Dental Check-ups**: Visit your dentist regularly for professional cleanings and check-ups. Be sure to inform your dentist that you have diabetes so they can provide extra care and monitor for signs of gum disease.
- **Hydration**: Drink plenty of water to help prevent dry mouth and keep your mouth hydrated. Avoid sugary drinks and snacks that can increase the risk of cavities and gum disease.

CONCLUSION

Preventing complications from diabetes requires a proactive approach to your health. Regular screenings, early detection of issues, and consistent management of blood sugar levels are crucial in reducing the risk of complications such as heart disease, neuropathy, kidney damage, and eye problems. Proper foot care and maintaining good oral hygiene are also essential components of a comprehensive diabetes management plan. By being vigilant, making informed choices, and working closely with your healthcare team, you can significantly reduce the risk of complications and improve your quality of life with diabetes.

CHAPTER 14: INNOVATIONS IN DIABETES CARE

The landscape of diabetes care is rapidly evolving, thanks to advancements in technology and research. With new tools, therapies, and innovations emerging, managing diabetes is becoming more precise, convenient, and effective. This chapter will explore the latest innovations in diabetes care, including advances in glucose monitoring, insulin delivery, diabetes management apps, and promising future treatments that could revolutionize the way we manage and treat diabetes.

---

1. EMERGING TECHNOLOGIES IN DIABETES CARE

Over the past decade, the diabetes care field has seen incredible innovations that have made managing the condition more efficient and effective. These advancements offer greater precision in tracking blood sugar levels, enhancing insulin delivery, and improving overall diabetes management.

1.1 GLUCOSE MONITORING TECHNOLOGIES

Traditionally, blood glucose monitoring required fingerstick tests, which could be inconvenient and painful. Now, there are more advanced methods that provide continuous, real-time data on glucose levels:

- CONTINUOUS GLUCOSE MONITORS (CGMS): CGMs are devices that measure blood sugar levels continuously throughout the day and night, providing real-time data on trends and patterns. This technology uses a small sensor inserted under the skin to measure glucose levels in the interstitial fluid (fluid between the cells). CGMs send the information to a device (such as a smartphone or receiver), allowing users to see their glucose levels in real-time, get alerts if levels are too high or too low, and make adjustments accordingly.

- FLASH GLUCOSE MONITORS: These are similar to CGMs but require the user to scan a sensor on their skin with a reader or smartphone app to get glucose readings. Flash monitors are more affordable than CGMs and offer a simpler alternative for those who don't need continuous monitoring.

- NON-INVASIVE GLUCOSE MONITORING: Several companies are working on developing non-invasive glucose monitors that do not require needles or sensors inserted under the skin. These devices are still in the research and development phase but could significantly change the future of diabetes care.

1.2 INSULIN DELIVERY SYSTEMS

Advances in insulin delivery systems have improved the accuracy and ease of insulin administration for people with diabetes. The two main innovations are insulin pumps and insulin pens, but there are also newer technologies that are paving the way for even more convenience.

- INSULIN PUMPS: Insulin pumps are small, wearable devices that deliver a continuous supply of insulin throughout the day via a small catheter inserted under the skin. They mimic the way a healthy pancreas releases insulin and can be programmed to deliver different amounts of insulin based on meals, activity, and glucose readings. Some insulin pumps are integrated with CGMs, allowing for automated adjustments in insulin delivery.
- CLOSED-LOOP SYSTEMS (ARTIFICIAL PANCREAS): The closed-loop system combines an insulin pump with a CGM to create an "artificial pancreas." This system automatically adjusts insulin delivery based on real-time glucose readings, reducing the need for manual insulin injections and allowing for tighter glucose control.
- INSULIN PENS: While insulin pens have been available for years, newer smart insulin pens have been developed that can track the time and amount of insulin administered, provide reminders for doses, and sync with diabetes management apps for better tracking.

1.3 DIABETES MANAGEMENT APPS

With the advent of smartphones, managing diabetes has become more streamlined through various apps that track blood sugar levels, meals, exercise, and medication. These apps offer a wealth of features designed to make diabetes care easier and more personalized.

- **BLOOD SUGAR TRACKERS:** Many apps now integrate with glucose meters or CGMs, allowing users to automatically log their blood sugar readings. These apps can track trends over time, helping users understand how their daily habits impact their blood sugar levels.

- **MEAL AND CARBOHYDRATE TRACKERS:** Apps that allow users to track their food intake, including carbohydrates, are becoming more sophisticated. Some apps have extensive food databases and can help users plan balanced meals while offering insulin dose recommendations based on the meal composition.

- **EXERCISE AND ACTIVITY TRACKING:** Many diabetes management apps include fitness trackers or integrate with wearables to monitor physical activity. By tracking exercise and offering insights into how physical activity affects blood sugar levels, these apps help users make better lifestyle decisions.

- **TELEMEDICINE:** Some apps also offer telehealth features, allowing users to consult with healthcare providers remotely, review their management plan, and receive advice on managing their diabetes.

---

2. THE FUTURE OF DIABETES TREATMENT

While current advancements are exciting, the future of diabetes treatment holds even more promise. With ongoing research, new therapies are on the horizon that could dramatically improve the quality of life for those with diabetes, and even potentially lead to cures.

2.1 ADVANCES IN DIABETES RESEARCH

- **Gene Therapy**: Research into gene therapy aims to treat diabetes by modifying genes to produce insulin-producing cells or restore insulin sensitivity. While this approach is still in its early stages, studies are showing potential in improving the function of the pancreas and reducing or eliminating the need for insulin therapy.
- **Beta Cell Regeneration**: One area of research focuses on regenerating the insulin-producing beta cells in the pancreas. In Type 1 diabetes, these cells are destroyed by the immune system, and restoring or regenerating these cells could provide a long-term solution. Researchers are exploring various methods, including stem cell therapy, to help the body produce more beta cells.
- **Immunotherapy for Type 1 Diabetes**: Type 1 diabetes is an autoimmune disease where the body attacks its own insulin-producing cells. Immunotherapy, which targets the immune system to stop this attack, is being explored as a potential treatment to preserve beta cells in newly diagnosed individuals.

- **Artificial Pancreas Improvements**: The development of closed-loop systems continues to progress, with newer systems becoming more sophisticated. Future iterations could include fully automated insulin delivery with no need for user intervention, improving diabetes management with even more precision.

2.2 POTENTIAL CURES FOR DIABETES

While there is no cure for diabetes at present, ongoing research brings hope for the future:

- **Stem Cell Therapy**: Stem cell research holds promise for creating insulin-producing cells in the lab, which could then be transplanted into the body to replace the damaged or non-functioning beta cells in the pancreas.
- **Islet Cell Transplantation**: For people with Type 1 diabetes, islet cell transplantation involves transplanting healthy insulin-producing cells from a donor pancreas into the recipient's liver. This procedure is still experimental but has shown promise in some cases. Future improvements in immunosuppressive drugs could make this option more accessible.
- **Gene Editing (CRISPR Technology)**: Gene editing technologies like CRISPR are being investigated as a way to "fix" the genetic mutations that cause Type 1 diabetes or increase the body's insulin production.

This field is still in the experimental stages but has the potential to revolutionize the treatment and possibly even cure diabetes in the future.

2.3 NEW TREATMENT OPTIONS

In addition to advances in potential cures, new treatments are being developed that may improve diabetes management:

- **SGLT-2 Inhibitors**: These medications help the kidneys remove excess glucose from the body through urine. They are showing promise in reducing blood sugar levels and improving heart and kidney health in people with diabetes.
- **GLP-1 Receptor Agonists**: These drugs work by mimicking the effects of a hormone that helps regulate blood sugar levels. GLP-1 receptor agonists can help reduce blood sugar and aid in weight loss, making them a helpful addition to diabetes treatment.
- **Smart Insulin**: Researchers are developing insulin that can "sense" blood sugar levels and adjust its action accordingly. This could further automate insulin delivery, reducing the need for constant monitoring and adjustment.

The future of diabetes care is bright, thanks to rapid advancements in technology and ongoing research. From continuous glucose monitors and insulin pumps to potential cures through gene therapy and stem cells, the tools available to those with diabetes are becoming increasingly sophisticated. By staying informed about these innovations, individuals with diabetes can take advantage of new technologies and treatments to improve their quality of life and manage their condition more effectively. As research continues, we may one day see a world where diabetes is no longer a lifelong condition, but a manageable aspect of a person's health with even greater hope for a cure.

Chapter 15: Long-Term Health and Wellness

Managing diabetes is a lifelong commitment, and as you age, it's essential to adapt your management plan to meet your evolving needs. This chapter focuses on strategies for maintaining health as you age with diabetes, adjusting your management plan over time, and staying informed about the latest research and guidelines.

---

1. Healthy Aging with Diabetes

As you age, managing diabetes can become more complex due to changes in your body's metabolism, increased risk of other health conditions, and the possibility of reduced physical activity. However, with the right approach, it's possible to maintain good health and live a long, fulfilling life with diabetes. Here are some strategies to help you age healthily while managing your condition:

1.1 Prioritizing Heart Health

People with diabetes are at increased risk for heart disease. To support your cardiovascular health as you age, focus on:

- **Maintaining a healthy diet**: Emphasize heart-healthy foods such as fruits, vegetables, whole grains, lean proteins, and healthy fats (e.g., omega-3 fatty acids found in fish).

- **Regular exercise**: Engage in aerobic exercise to improve circulation and heart health. Activities like walking, swimming, or cycling can help maintain heart function and reduce the risk of cardiovascular disease.

- **Managing blood pressure and cholesterol**: Regularly monitor your blood pressure and cholesterol levels, as these factors also contribute to heart disease. Medications, if necessary, should be taken as prescribed.

1.2 MAINTAINING MOBILITY AND INDEPENDENCE

As you age, physical changes like reduced strength, joint pain, or limited flexibility can affect your ability to perform daily tasks. Managing diabetes and staying active can help prevent or delay these issues:

- **Exercise for strength and balance**: Incorporate strength training exercises to maintain muscle mass and balance exercises to prevent falls. These can be as simple as bodyweight exercises, resistance bands, or light weights.

- **Flexibility exercises**: Stretching, yoga, or Pilates can improve flexibility and reduce stiffness, making it easier to move and stay independent.

- **Pain management**: For those experiencing joint pain or other discomforts related to diabetes, work with your healthcare team to explore pain management options that are compatible with your diabetes treatment plan.

1.3 MENTAL AND COGNITIVE HEALTH

Cognitive decline and mental health issues, such as depression or anxiety, can become more prevalent as you age, particularly in individuals with diabetes. To support mental wellness:

- **Stay mentally active**: Engage in activities that stimulate your brain, such as reading, puzzles, or learning new skills.
- **Manage stress**: Practice relaxation techniques like deep breathing, meditation, or mindfulness to reduce stress levels.
- **Seek support**: If you experience feelings of depression or anxiety, it's important to seek professional support. Therapy, medication, or support groups can help you manage mental health effectively.

1.4 SKIN AND FOOT CARE

Diabetes increases the risk of skin and foot problems due to poor circulation and neuropathy. Here are ways to protect your skin and feet:

- **Daily foot inspections**: Check your feet every day for cuts, blisters, sores, or infections. Diabetes-related nerve damage may reduce your ability to feel pain, so regular foot exams are essential.
- **Skin protection**: Keep your skin hydrated and avoid harsh chemicals that can cause irritation. Consider using gentle, fragrance-free moisturizers and avoid hot showers or baths, which can dry out the skin.

---

2. ADAPTING YOUR MANAGEMENT PLAN OVER TIME

As you age, your health needs change, and it's important to adapt your diabetes management plan to reflect those changes. Regular consultations with your healthcare team are key to adjusting your approach.

2.1 CHANGES IN BLOOD SUGAR TARGETS

As you age, your body may respond differently to insulin and medications, and your blood sugar targets may need to be adjusted. Factors such as changes in physical activity, weight, meal patterns, and other health conditions can influence your blood sugar levels. Work with your healthcare provider to set realistic blood sugar goals based on your age, health status, and lifestyle.

2.2 ADJUSTING MEDICATIONS

Some medications may become less effective as you age or may interact with other medications you are taking for age-related conditions. It's important to:

- **Review medications regularly**: Periodically review all medications with your healthcare provider to ensure they are still necessary and safe for you. Adjust dosages or switch to different medications if needed.
- **Explore new treatment options**: New medications or treatments may become available that are better suited for older adults. Stay open to exploring these options to improve your diabetes management.

2.3 MANAGING MULTIPLE HEALTH CONDITIONS

Older adults with diabetes often have additional health conditions, such as high blood pressure, arthritis, or osteoporosis. Coordinating care between specialists and managing multiple conditions can be complex, so:

- **Coordinate care**: Work closely with your healthcare team to ensure that all your health conditions are managed effectively and that treatments don't interfere with each other.
- **Monitor for complications**: Regular screenings for diabetes-related complications such as kidney disease, neuropathy, and eye problems are critical in older adults. Early detection can help prevent or delay the progression of complications.

2.4 ADJUSTING LIFESTYLE CHOICES

Your physical abilities, energy levels, and preferences may change as you age. This means your exercise and nutrition plans may need adjustments:

- **Modify exercise routines**: Choose low-impact exercises, such as walking, swimming, or gentle yoga, to accommodate changes in mobility and stamina.
- **Reevaluate your diet**: Ensure your meals are well-balanced and meet your nutritional needs. You may need to adjust portions, increase fiber intake, or explore new eating patterns to maintain blood sugar control.

---

3. STAYING INFORMED

Staying up-to-date with the latest diabetes research, treatment options, and health recommendations is crucial for managing your condition effectively over time.

3.1 KEEP LEARNING ABOUT DIABETES

Diabetes research is constantly evolving, and new treatments, tools, and techniques emerge regularly. Staying informed about the latest findings will help you make the best decisions for your health:

- **Attend diabetes education programs**: Many healthcare organizations offer diabetes education programs that can help you stay informed and better manage your condition.
- **Read reputable resources**: Follow trusted sources like the American Diabetes Association, the Centers for Disease Control and Prevention (CDC), and diabetes-focused medical journals for updates on research and recommendations.

3.2 REGULAR CHECK-UPS

Regular check-ups with your healthcare team are essential to ensuring your diabetes management is on track. These check-ups allow for:

- **Ongoing monitoring**: Regular tests like A1C, kidney function, and eye exams help detect complications early.
- **Personalized advice**: As your body changes, your healthcare provider can give you specific advice tailored to your evolving needs.

3.3 EMBRACE NEW TECHNOLOGIES

With emerging technologies, managing diabetes is becoming easier and more effective. Stay informed about new glucose monitoring systems, insulin delivery devices, diabetes management apps, and other innovations that could improve your daily management of the condition.

CONCLUSION

Living with diabetes as you age doesn't mean compromising your quality of life. By adapting your management plan, focusing on maintaining overall health, and staying informed about the latest developments in diabetes care, you can continue to live a fulfilling and healthy life. Regular consultations with your healthcare team, staying active, eating well, and monitoring your health are key components of successful long-term diabetes management. Aging with diabetes is a journey, but with the right approach, you can thrive and enjoy your later years with good health and vitality.

Final Thoughts

Managing diabetes is an ongoing journey that requires commitment, flexibility, and an informed approach. Throughout this book, we've explored the vital aspects of living well with diabetes, from understanding the science behind the condition to developing a comprehensive management plan that includes nutrition, exercise, medication, and emotional well-being. The ultimate goal is not just to manage diabetes, but to thrive and maintain a high quality of life despite the challenges the condition may bring.

Empowerment Through Knowledge

Knowledge is one of the most powerful tools you can use to take control of your health. By learning about diabetes, its impact on the body, and the latest treatment options, you empower yourself to make informed decisions that align with your health goals. Understanding the importance of blood sugar control, how medications work, and the ways to manage stress and maintain mental well-being will help you feel confident in managing your condition.

You have the ability to shape your future with diabetes. Every small step toward healthier choices—whether it's adjusting your diet, staying active, monitoring your blood sugar, or seeking emotional support—will add up to meaningful progress. Empowerment comes from knowing that you can oversee your health, even when faced with challenges.

THE IMPORTANCE OF ONGOING MANAGEMENT

Diabetes management is not a one-time fix; it is a continuous process that requires regular monitoring, adjustments, and self-care. As your body changes, so do your diabetes management needs. That's why ongoing engagement with your healthcare team, staying informed about new research, and making adjustments to your treatment plan are essential.

Regular check-ups, consistent blood sugar monitoring, and lifestyle management are key to preventing complications and ensuring long-term well-being. Just as importantly, maintaining a positive and proactive mindset toward managing your condition can make all the difference in living a fulfilling life with diabetes.

By taking an active role in your diabetes management and embracing the tools, resources, and knowledge available, you are not just surviving with diabetes—you are thriving. With the right approach and mindset, you can live a long, healthy, and active life, fully in control of your health and well-being.

Remember: You are stronger than your diagnosis. With the right support and mindset, you can continue to manage diabetes effectively and live your life to the fullest. Keep learning, stay motivated, and never stop advocating for your health.

GLOSSARY OF TERMS

- **A1C (Hemoglobin A1C):** A blood test that measures your average blood glucose level over the past 2 to 3 months. It is used to diagnose and monitor diabetes.
- **Carbohydrates:** Nutrients found in food that provide energy, which can affect blood sugar levels. Carbs include sugars, starches, and fibers.
- **Insulin:** A hormone produced by the pancreas that allows glucose (sugar) to enter cells for energy. In diabetes, the body either doesn't produce enough insulin (Type 1) or doesn't use it effectively (Type 2).
- **Glycemic Index (GI):** A ranking of how carbohydrate-containing foods affect blood glucose levels. Foods with a high GI cause a rapid increase in blood sugar.
- **Continuous Glucose Monitor (CGM):** A device that continuously measures blood glucose levels throughout the day and night.
- **Hypoglycemia:** Low blood sugar levels, often caused by too much insulin or insufficient food.
- **Hyperglycemia:** High blood sugar levels, commonly caused by insufficient insulin or improper management of diabetes.

- **Prediabetes:** A condition where blood sugar levels are higher than normal but not high enough to be classified as diabetes.

- **Type 1 Diabetes:** An autoimmune condition where the body doesn't produce insulin, requiring insulin therapy.

- **Type 2 Diabetes:** A condition where the body doesn't use insulin properly (insulin resistance), and the pancreas can't keep up with the demand for insulin.

Websites:

- **American Diabetes Association (ADA):** www.diabetes.org - Offers a wealth of information about diabetes care, research, and living with the condition.

- **Centers for Disease Control and Prevention (CDC) – Diabetes:** www.cdc.gov/diabetes - Provides facts on diabetes prevention, management, and complications.

- **Diabetes UK:** www.diabetes.org.uk - Offers resources for those living with diabetes in the UK, including advice, research, and support.

- **"The Diabetes Cookbook" by the American Diabetes Association:** A comprehensive guide to meal planning for those with diabetes.
- **"Think Like a Pancreas" by Gary Scheiner:** A practical guide to understanding insulin therapy and managing Type 1 and Type 2 diabetes.
- **"The Diabetes Solution" by Dr. Jorge Rodriguez:** A comprehensive guide for managing diabetes through diet and lifestyle changes.

SUPPORT GROUPS:

- **Diabetes Support Groups at Local Hospitals:** Many hospitals offer in-person or virtual support groups.
- **Online Diabetes Communities:** Websites like Reddit's r/diabetes or Facebook groups provide emotional support and advice from peers.

DIABETES MANAGEMENT CHECKLIST

Daily Tasks:

- Monitor blood glucose levels as prescribed.
- Take medications or insulin as directed.
- Eat balanced meals, focusing on controlling carbohydrate intake.

- Engage in at least 30 minutes of physical activity.

- Stay hydrated, avoiding sugary drinks.

- Check feet for any signs of damage or infection.

- Record food intake and exercise to track patterns.

WEEKLY TASKS:

- Review blood glucose logs with your healthcare team.

- Plan and prep meals for the upcoming week.

- Exercise at least three times per week (strength training, cardio, or a mix).

- Monitor for any signs of stress, illness, or complications.

- Inspect your skin for cuts or infections, especially on the feet.

MONTHLY TASKS:

- Schedule check-ups with your healthcare provider.

- Review A1C levels and blood pressure with your doctor.

- Evaluate and adjust medications as needed.

- Track your weight and discuss any changes with your healthcare team.

- Review your diabetes care plan for any necessary updates.

30-Day Diabetes-Friendly Meal Plan

This meal plan focuses on nutrient-dense foods, low glycemic index carbs, and plenty of fiber to help manage blood sugar levels while promoting overall health. You can adjust portion sizes and food choices based on individual preferences and specific dietary needs. Always consult with a healthcare professional or dietitian to personalize your meal plan further.

Week 1:

Day 1:

Breakfast: Scrambled eggs with spinach and tomatoes, whole-grain toast

Lunch: Grilled chicken salad with avocado, mixed greens, and olive oil dressing

Dinner: Baked salmon with roasted Brussels sprouts and quinoa

Snack: Greek yogurt with almonds

Day 2:

Breakfast: Oatmeal with chia seeds, walnuts, and blueberries

Lunch: Turkey and avocado wrap in whole-wheat tortilla

Dinner: Stir-fried tofu with mixed vegetables and brown rice

Snack: A handful of mixed nuts

Day 3:

Breakfast: Smoothie with spinach, almond milk, protein powder, and berries

Lunch: Lentil soup with side salad (olive oil dressing)

Dinner: Grilled chicken breast, baked sweet potato, steamed broccoli

Snack: Carrot sticks with hummus

DAY 4:

Breakfast: Greek yogurt with cinnamon, flaxseeds, and raspberries

Lunch: Quinoa chickpea salad with lemon-olive oil dressing

Dinner: Baked cod with sautéed spinach and roasted cauliflower

Snack: Sunflower seeds

DAY 5:

Breakfast: Whole-grain toast with avocado, poached egg, and chia seeds

Lunch: Grilled shrimp salad with mixed greens, avocado, and olive oil dressing

Dinner: Turkey meatballs with zucchini noodles and marinara sauce

Snack: Apple with almond butter

DAY 6:

Breakfast: Scrambled eggs with bell peppers, onions, and spinach

Lunch: Grilled chicken, roasted butternut squash, and green beans

Dinner: Beef stir-fry with broccoli, bell peppers, and cauliflower rice

Snack: Sliced cucumber and cherry tomatoes with hummus

DAY 7:

Breakfast: Chia pudding with almond milk, chia seeds, and strawberries

Lunch: Tuna salad with mixed greens and olive oil dressing

Dinner: Grilled chicken with roasted carrots and kale

Snack: Walnuts and a small piece of dark chocolate

DAY 8:

Breakfast: Scrambled eggs with mushrooms and spinach, whole-grain toast

Lunch: Quinoa and chickpea salad with cucumber, tomatoes, and lemon dressing

Dinner: Baked salmon with asparagus and roasted sweet potatoes

Snack: Greek yogurt with a few almonds

DAY 9:

Breakfast: Oatmeal with flaxseeds, blueberries, and walnuts

Lunch: Grilled turkey and avocado salad with olive oil dressing

Dinner: Stir-fried chicken with broccoli, bell peppers, and brown rice

Snack: Mixed nuts

DAY 10:

Breakfast: Smoothie with unsweetened almond milk, protein powder, and spinach

Lunch: Lentil soup with a side of mixed greens salad

Dinner: Grilled shrimp with zucchini noodles and side of roasted cauliflower

Snack: Carrot sticks with hummus

DAY 11:

Breakfast: Greek yogurt with cinnamon, chia seeds, and strawberries

Lunch: Grilled chicken breast with roasted Brussels sprouts and quinoa

Dinner: Baked cod with roasted broccoli and sweet potato

Snack: A handful of sunflower seeds

DAY 12:

Breakfast: Avocado toast with poached eggs and chia seeds

Lunch: Grilled shrimp salad with avocado, cucumber, and mixed greens

Dinner: Beef stir-fry with mixed vegetables and cauliflower rice

Snack: Apple with almond butter

DAY 13:

Breakfast: Scrambled eggs with spinach, onions, and tomatoes

Lunch: Grilled chicken with roasted butternut squash and green beans

Dinner: Baked chicken breast with quinoa and steamed broccoli

Snack: Cucumber slices with hummus

DAY 14:

Breakfast: Chia pudding with almond milk, chia seeds, and raspberries

Lunch: Tuna salad with avocado and mixed greens

Dinner: Grilled salmon with roasted cauliflower and a side of kale

Snack: Walnuts and dark chocolate

WEEK 3:

DAY 15:

Breakfast: Scrambled eggs with mushrooms, spinach, and bell peppers

Lunch: Quinoa and chickpea salad with mixed greens and olive oil dressing

Dinner: Grilled chicken with roasted Brussels sprouts and sweet potato

Snack: Greek yogurt with a few almonds

Breakfast: Oatmeal with chia seeds, flaxseeds, and blueberries

Lunch: Turkey and avocado wrap in whole-wheat tortilla

Dinner: Stir-fried tofu with broccoli, carrots, and brown rice

Snack: Mixed nuts

DAY 17:

Breakfast: Smoothie with spinach, almond milk, chia seeds, and protein powder

Lunch: Lentil soup with side salad (olive oil dressing)

Dinner: Grilled chicken breast, quinoa, and steamed green beans

Snack: Carrot sticks with hummus

DAY 18:

Breakfast: Greek yogurt with cinnamon, raspberries, and flaxseeds

Lunch: Tuna salad with mixed greens and olive oil dressing

Dinner: Baked cod with sautéed spinach and roasted cauliflower

Snack: Sunflower seeds

DAY 19:

Breakfast: Avocado toast with poached eggs and chia seeds

Lunch: Grilled shrimp with mixed greens, avocado, and olive oil dressing

Dinner: Turkey meatballs with zucchini noodles and marinara sauce

Snack: Apple with almond butter

DAY 20:

Breakfast: Scrambled eggs with onions, spinach, and bell peppers

Lunch: Grilled chicken with roasted carrots and green beans

Dinner: Beef stir-fry with broccoli, bell peppers, and cauliflower rice

Snack: Sliced cucumber and cherry tomatoes with hummus

DAY 21:

Breakfast: Chia pudding with almond milk, chia seeds, and strawberries

Lunch: Quinoa chickpea salad with cucumber, tomatoes, and lemon dressing

Dinner: Grilled salmon with roasted sweet potato and kale

Snack: Walnuts and dark chocolate

WEEK 4:

DAY 22:

Breakfast: Scrambled eggs with spinach and tomatoes, whole-grain toast

Lunch: Grilled chicken salad with avocado, mixed greens, and olive oil dressing

Dinner: Baked salmon with roasted Brussels sprouts and quinoa

Snack: Greek yogurt with almonds

DAY 23:

Breakfast: Oatmeal with chia seeds, walnuts, and blueberries

Lunch: Turkey and avocado wrap in whole-wheat tortilla

Dinner: Stir-fried tofu with mixed vegetables and brown rice

Snack: A handful of mixed nuts

DAY 24:

Breakfast: Smoothie with spinach, almond milk, protein powder, and berries

Lunch: Lentil soup with side salad (olive oil dressing)

Dinner: Grilled chicken breast, baked sweet potato, steamed broccoli

Snack: Carrot sticks with hummus

DAY 25:

Breakfast: Greek yogurt with cinnamon, flaxseeds, and raspberries

Lunch: Quinoa chickpea salad with lemon-olive oil dressing

Dinner: Baked cod with sautéed spinach and roasted cauliflower

Snack: Sunflower seeds

DAY 26:

Breakfast: Whole-grain toast with avocado, poached egg, and chia seeds

Lunch: Grilled shrimp salad with mixed greens, avocado, and olive oil dressing

Dinner: Turkey meatballs with zucchini noodles and marinara sauce

Snack: Apple with almond butter

DAY 27:

Breakfast: Scrambled eggs with bell peppers, onions, and spinach

Lunch: Grilled chicken, roasted butternut squash, and green beans

Dinner: Beef stir-fry with broccoli, bell peppers, and cauliflower rice

Snack: Sliced cucumber and cherry tomatoes with hummus

DAY 28:

Breakfast: Chia pudding with almond milk, chia seeds, and strawberries

Lunch: Tuna salad with avocado and mixed greens

Dinner: Grilled chicken with roasted carrots and kale

Snack: Walnuts and dark chocolate

Breakfast: Scrambled eggs with mushrooms and spinach, whole-grain toast

Lunch: Quinoa and chickpea salad with cucumber, tomatoes, and lemon dressing

Dinner: Baked salmon with roasted sweet potatoes and broccoli

Snack: Greek yogurt with almonds

Day 30:

Breakfast: Oatmeal with flaxseeds, blueberries, and walnuts

Lunch: Grilled turkey and avocado salad with olive oil dressing

Dinner: Stir-fried chicken with broccoli, bell peppers, and brown rice

Snack: Mixed nuts

GENERAL GUIDELINES:

- **Hydration**: Aim for at least 8 cups of water per day. Herbal teas are a great option too.
- **Portion Sizes**: Be mindful of portion sizes, particularly with starchy vegetables, grains, and fruits, to help control blood sugar levels.
- **Snack Wisely**: Choose snacks that combine protein, fiber, and healthy fats to keep you feeling satisfied and prevent blood sugar spikes.

Date	Type of Exercise	Duration	Intensity	Blood Sugar Before	Blood Sugar After	Notes
2024-12-01	Walking	30 min	Moderate	150 mg/dL	120 mg/dL	Felt energized
2024-12-02	Strength Training	45 min	High	170 mg/dL	160 mg/dL	Slightly fatigued
2024-12-03	Swimming	40 min	Moderate	160 mg/dL	140 mg/dL	No issues during
2024-12-04	Yoga	30 min	Low	140 mg/dL	130 mg/dL	Felt relaxed

Use this log to track your physical activity and its effects on blood sugar levels, which can help identify trends and adjust your management plan accordingly.

1. **American Diabetes Association (ADA).** (2021). *Standards of Medical Care in Diabetes—2021.* Diabetes Care, 44(Supplement 1), S1-S2. https://doi.org/10.2337/dc21-S001

     o   A comprehensive set of guidelines and recommendations from the ADA for the diagnosis, treatment, and management of diabetes.

2. **Centers for Disease Control and Prevention (CDC).** (2020). *National Diabetes Statistics Report, 2020.* U.S. Department of Health and Human Services.

     https://www.cdc.gov/diabetes/library/reports/reportcard.html

     o   A detailed report on the prevalence, risk factors, and impact of diabetes in the United States.

3. **Scheiner, G. (2011).** *Think Like a Pancreas: A Practical Guide to Managing Diabetes with Insulin.* 3rd Edition. Torrey Pines Press.

     o   A practical guide on insulin management for individuals with Type 1 and Type 2 diabetes.

4. **Rodriguez, J. (2013).** *The Diabetes Solution: The Small Carb Diabetes Diet That Can Save Your Life.* Harper Collins.

     o   A book outlining a structured approach to diabetes management through diet and lifestyle changes.

5. **Diabetes UK.** (2019). *Diabetes: What You Need to Know.* Diabètes UK.

     https://www.diabetes.org.uk

- A comprehensive resource on living with diabetes, including diet, exercise, medication, and emotional well-being.

6. **Mayo Clinic.** (2020). *Diabetes: Complications.* Mayo Clinic. https://www.mayoclinic.org/diseases-conditions/diabetes/complications

    - A thorough overview of the complications that can arise from uncontrolled diabetes and prevention strategies.

7. **National Institute of Diabetes and Digestive and Kidney Diseases (NIDDK).** (2020). *Managing Diabetes.* https://www.niddk.nih.gov/health-information/diabetes

    - A trusted source of information from the NIH about managing diabetes, including medications, blood sugar monitoring, and lifestyle changes.

8. **American Diabetes Association (ADA).** (2020). *The Glycemic Index and Blood Sugar Control.* Diabetes Forecast. https://www.diabetesforecast.org/

    - A journal article explaining the role of the glycemic index in managing blood sugar levels.

9. **Yancy, W. S., & Westman, E. C. (2014).** *Low-Carbohydrate Diets and Type 2 Diabetes: A Review of the Evidence.* The Journal of Clinical Endocrinology & Metabolism, 99(11), 4310–4317. https://doi.org/10.1210/jc.2014-3054

- o An exploration of the impact of low-carb diets on Type 2 diabetes management, focusing on evidence-based results.

10. **World Health Organization (WHO).** (2016). *Global Report on Diabetes.* WHO Press. https://www.who.int/diabetes/global-report

   - o A global overview of diabetes prevalence, risk factors, and strategic goals for managing the global diabetes epidemic.

11. **Stenholm, S., et al. (2018).** *Sleep Duration and Its Association with Diabetes Risk and Management.* Diabetes Research and Clinical Practice, 146, 48-55. https://doi.org/10.1016/j.diabres.2018.10.014

   - o A study examining the link between sleep duration, blood sugar control, and diabetes risk.

12. **American Heart Association.** (2020). *Diabetes and Cardiovascular Disease.* https://www.heart.org

   - o A resource outlining the connection between diabetes and heart disease, and how to manage both conditions effectively.

13. **National Institutes of Health (NIH).** (2021). *Prevention of Type 2 Diabetes.* https://www.niddk.nih.gov/health-information/diabetes/prevention

   - o Information on risk reduction and prevention strategies for Type 2 diabetes, including lifestyle modifications and medications.

14. **American Academy of Sleep Medicine.** (2019). *Sleep Apnea and Diabetes.* Sleep Medicine Reviews, 45, 72-77. https://doi.org/10.1016/j.smrv.2018.02.001

- A review article discussing the relationship between sleep apnea and diabetes, with emphasis on management techniques.

15. **The Diabetes Control and Complications Trial (DCCT).** (1993). *The Effect of Intensive Diabetes Therapy on the Development and Progression of Long-Term Complications in Insulin-Dependent Diabetes Mellitus.* The New England Journal of Medicine, 329(14), 977-986. https://doi.org/10.1056/NEJM199309303291401

- Landmark study examining the benefits of tight blood glucose control on the prevention of diabetes complications.

These references provide the foundation for the information in this book, drawing on trusted resources from healthcare organizations, studies, and expert literature to provide accurate and up-to-date insights for diabetes management.

The inspiration for writing this book came from the fact I have suffered with type 2 diabetes for a few years and did not know how to manage her health. The growing prevalence of diabetes, many people still lack clear, accessible, and actionable information to effectively manage the condition. I saw that individuals living with diabetes often feel overwhelmed by conflicting advice and complex medical terminology. This book is designed to serve as a comprehensive, yet easy-to-understand resource that helps individuals and their families take charge of their health and make informed decisions every day.

Understanding that diabetes is not just a medical condition but a lifestyle that affects every aspect of life. I aim to empower readers by providing a holistic approach to diabetes management—incorporating diet, exercise, emotional well-being, and medical care. Through this book, I hope to inspire confidence in those living with diabetes, offering them the tools and knowledge they need to thrive and live a fulfilling life.